# Nonmalignant Hematology

*Guest Editor*

ROBERT I. PARKER, MD

# CRITICAL CARE CLINICS

www.criticalcare.theclinics.com

*Consulting Editor*
RICHARD W. CARLSON, MD, PhD

July 2012 • Volume 28 • Number 3

SAUNDERS an imprint of ELSEVIER, Inc.

**W.B. SAUNDERS COMPANY**
*A Division of Elsevier Inc.*

Elsevier Inc. • 1600 John F. Kennedy Blvd., • Suite 1800 • Philadelphia, Pennsylvania 19103-2899

http://www.theclinics.com

**CRITICAL CARE CLINICS Volume 28, Number 3**
**July 2012 ISSN 0749-0704, ISBN-13: 978-1-4557-4937-9**

Editor: Patrick Manley
Developmental Editor: Donald Mumford

*Critical Care Clinics* (ISSN: 0749-0704) is published quarterly by Elsevier Inc., 360 Park Avenue South, New York, NY 10010-1710. Months of issue are January, April, July, and October. Business and Editorial Offices: 1600 John F. Kennedy Blvd., Suite 1800, Philadelphia, PA 19103-2899. Customer Service Office: 6277 Sea Harbor Drive, Orlando, FL 32887-4800. Periodicals postage paid at New York, NY and additional mailing offices. Subscription prices are $193.00 per year for US individuals, $463.00 per year for US institution, $94.00 per year for US students and residents, $238.00 per year for Canadian individuals, $574.00 per year for Canadian institutions, $278.00 per year for international individuals, $574.00 per year for international institutions and $137.00 per year for Canadian and foreign students/residents. To receive student/resident rate, orders must be accompanied by name of affiliated institution, date of term, and the signature of program/residency coordinator on institution letterhead. Orders will be billed at individual rate until proof of status is received. Foreign air speed delivery is included in all *Clinics* subscription prices. All prices are subject to change without notice. POSTMASTER: Send address changes to *Critical Care Clinics*, Elsevier Periodicals Customer Service, 11830 Westline Industrial Drive, St. Louis, MO 63146. **Customer Service: 1-800-654-2452 (US). From outside of the US, call 1-314-447-8871. Fax: 1-314-447-8029. E-mail: journalscustomerservice-usa@elsevier.com (for print support) or journalsonlinesupport-usa@elsevier.com (for online support).**

*Reprints.* For copies of 100 or more of articles in this publication, please contact the Commercial Reprints Department, Elsevier Inc., 360 Park Avenue South, New York, NY 10010-1710. Tel.: 212-633-3813; Fax: 212-462-1935; E-mail: reprints@elsevier.com.

*Critical Care Clinics* is also published in Spanish by Editorial Inter-Medica, Junin 917, 1$^{er}$ A, 1113, Buenos Aires, Argentina.

*Critical Care Clinics* is covered in *MEDLINE/PubMed (Index Medicus), EMBASE/Excerpta Medica, Current Concepts/Clinical Medicine, ISI/BIOMED,* and *Chemical Abstracts.*

Printed and bound by CPI Group (UK) Ltd, Croydon, CR0 4YY

Transferred to Digital Print 2012

# Contributors

## CONSULTING EDITOR

**RICHARD W. CARLSON, MD, PhD**
Chairman Emeritus, Department of Medicine, Maricopa Medical Center; Director,
Medical Intensive Care Unit; Professor, University of Arizona College of Medicine;
Professor, Department of Medicine, Mayo Graduate School of Medicine, Phoenix,
Arizona

## GUEST EDITOR

**ROBERT I. PARKER, MD**
Professor and Vice Chair for Academic Affairs, Department of Pediatrics, Stony Brook
University School of Medicine; Director, Pediatric Hematology/Oncology, Stony Brook
Long Island Children's Hospital, Stony Brook, New York

## AUTHORS

**REBECCA BEYTH, MD, MSc**
Department of Medicine, University of Florida, College of Medicine, Health Science
Center, Gainesville, Florida

**JOSEPH A. CARCILLO, MD**
Departments of Critical Care Medicine and Pediatrics, University of Pittsburgh School of
Medicine, Pittsburgh, Pennsylvania

**MARK A. CROWTHER, MD, MSc, FRCPC**
Department of Medicine, McMaster University and St Joseph's Hospital, Hamilton,
Ontario, Canada

**KEVIN DASHER, MD**
Hepatology Fellow, Baylor University Medical Center, Dallas, Texas

**SATOSHI GANDO, MD, PhD, FCCM**
Division of Acute and Critical Care Medicine, Department of Anesthesiology and Critical
Care Medicine, Hokkaido University Graduate School of Medicine, Sapporo, Japan

**JORDANA R. GOLDMAN, MD**
Section of Critical Care Medicine, Department of Pediatrics, Baylor College of Medicine/
Texas Children's Hospital, Houston, Texas

**LAWRENCE TIM GOODNOUGH, MD**
Professor of Pathology and Medicine, Stanford University; Director of Transfusion
Services, Stanford University Medical Center, Stanford, California

**JOSEPH E. KISS, MD**
The Institute of Transfusion Medicine, Division of Hematology/Oncology, Department of
Medicine, University of Pittsburgh School of Medicine, Pittsburgh, Pennsylvania

**MARK R. LOONEY, MD**
Division of Pulmonary, Critical Care, Allergy and Sleep Medicine, Department of Medicine and Laboratory Medicine, University of California, San Francisco, San Francisco, California

**TRUNG C. NGUYEN, MD**
Assistant Professor, Section of Critical Care Medicine, Department of Pediatrics, Baylor College of Medicine/Texas Children's Hospital; Division of Thrombosis Research, Department of Medicine, Baylor College of Medicine, Houston, Texas

**ROBERT I. PARKER, MD**
Professor and Vice Chair for Academic Affairs, Department of Pediatrics, Stony Brook University School of Medicine; Director, Pediatric Hematology/Oncology, Stony Brook Long Island Children's Hospital, Stony Brook, New York

**MICHAEL PIAGNERELLI, MD, PhD**
Department of Intensive Care, CHU-Charleroi, Université Libre de Bruxelles, Charleroi, Belgium

**DEVINA PRAKASH, MBBS**
Clinical Associate Professor and Director, Sickle Cell Program, Division of Pediatric Hematology Oncology, Stony Brook Long Island Children's Hospital, Stony Brook, New York

**ANITA RAJASEKHAR, MD**
Department of Medicine, University of Florida, College of Medicine, Health Science Center, Gainesville, Florida

**DAVID M. SAYAH, MD, PhD**
Division of Pulmonary, Critical Care, Allergy and Sleep Medicine, Department of Medicine, University of California, San Francisco, San Francisco, California

**PEARL TOY, MD**
Department of Laboratory Medicine, University of California, San Francisco, San Francisco, California

**JAMES F. TROTTER, MD**
Medical Director of Liver Transplantation, Baylor University Medical Center, Dallas, Texas

**JEAN-LOUIS VINCENT, MD, PhD**
Professor and Head, Department of Intensive Care, Erasme Hospital, Université Libre de Bruxelles, Brussels, Belgium

# Contents

> Anemia is common in the ICU, increasing morbidity and mortality. Its etiology is multifactorial but anemia of inflammation is the most common cause, followed closely by iron deficiency. The two conditions often coexist and it can be difficult to diagnose iron deficiency in the context of anemia of inflammation. Blood transfusions and use of erythropoietin agonists are two modalities used to correct anemia in critically ill patients. Randomized controlled trials have not supported the use of either therapy except in well defined clinical situations. Better understanding of the pathophysiology of anemia of inflammation may lead to development of novel therapies.

> Anemia is common in critically ill patients, but treatment with red blood cell transfusions can have unwanted effects. Limiting the occurrence and severity of anemia by using erythropoietic agents (iron and/or recombinant erythropoietin), therefore, remains an attractive option during the intensive care unit stay but also after hospital discharge. Moreover, these agents may have additional beneficial properties. In this article the authors review the rationale for the administration of iron and/or erythropoietin in critically ill patients.

> Transfusion-related acute lung injury (TRALI) is the leading cause of transfusion-related mortality. TRALI presents as acute lung injury (ALI) within 6 hours after blood product transfusion. Diagnosing TRALI requires a high index of suspicion, and the exclusion of circulatory overload or other causes of ALI. The pathophysiology of TRALI is incompletely understood, but in part involves transfusion of certain anti-neutrophil antibodies, anti-HLA antibodies, or other bioactive substances, into susceptible recipients. Recent studies have identified both recipient and transfusion risk factors for the development of TRALI. This article describes these TRALI risk factors, as well as diagnosis, treatment and prevention strategies.

> Disseminated intravascular coagulation (DIC) is an acquired syndrome characterized by microvascular thrombosis resulting from systemic activation of coagulation, and it should be diagnosed and treated as early as possible. No single test is sufficiently accurate to establish or rule out a diagnosis of DIC. Therefore, diagnostic scoring uses a combination of several laboratory tests. Three diagnostic scoring systems are now available and validated. Because it is not easy to assess the superiority or inferiority of these scoring systems, it may be better to select the scoring system depending on the need for an early or affirmative diagnosis of DIC.

> Coagulopathy, one of the cardinal features of advanced liver disease, is related to multiple factors including impaired synthetic function, thrombocytopenia, excessive fibrinolysis, platelet dysfunction, and disseminated intravascular coagulopathy. In the intensive care unit, management of coagulopathy may require treatment, particularly in the actively bleeding patient or in preparation for invasive procedures. This article reviews the background of coagulopathy in patients with end-stage liver disease and management options and comments on common clinical scenarios.

> Thrombocytopenia is common in critically ill patients and increases morbidity and mortality. A diagnosis of heparin-induced thrombocytopenia (HIT) is frequently considered in any ICU patient who develops thrombocytopenia in the context of ongoing heparin exposure. As the usual tests to diagnose HIT are often neither specific nor sensitive enough to be confirmatory, the intensivist must largely rely on clinical judgment in treatment decisions. Patients in the ICU may also develop thrombocytopenia resulting from non-HIT immune mechanisms, nonimmune platelet consumption, and from decreased platelet production due to preexisting disorders or as a result of their critical illness and/or drug therapy.

> Plasma therapy and plasma products such as prothrombin complex concentrates (PCCs), and recombinant activated factor VII (rFVIIa) are

used in the setting of massive or refractory hemorrhage. Their roles have evolved because of newly emerging options, variable availability, and heterogeneity in guidelines. These factors can be attributable to lack of evidence-based support for a defined role for plasma therapy, variability in coagulation factor content among PCCs, and uncertainty regarding safety and efficacy of rFVIIa in these settings. This review summarizes these issues and provides insight regarding use of these options in management of refractory or massive bleeding.

## Newer Anticoagulants in Critically Ill Patients                                427

Anita Rajasekhar, Rebecca Beyth, and Mark A. Crowther

Critically ill patients are at increased risk for development of thrombosis. In addition, thrombosis is often unrecognized in this population. Furthermore, these patients are particularly susceptible to bleeding complications from anticoagulants. Herein the authors review the pharmacology, data from clinical trials, management of bleeding complications, and perioperative use of these agents in the intensive care unit population. Well-designed clinical trials are needed to improve our understanding of the safety and efficacy of these newer agents in critically ill patients.

## The Role of Plasmapheresis in Critical Illness                                453

Trung C. Nguyen, Joseph E. Kiss, Jordana R. Goldman, and Joseph A. Carcillo

In this article, the authors review the current recommendations from the American Society for Apheresis regarding the use of plasmapheresis in many of the diseases that intensivists commonly encounter in critically ill patients. Recent experience indicates that therapeutic plasma exchange may be useful in a wide spectrum of illnesses characterized by microvascular thrombosis, the presence of autoantibodies, immune activation with dysregulation of immune response, and some infections.

# CRITICAL CARE CLINICS

# Preface

# Hematologic Issues in the ICU

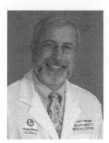

Robert I. Parker, MD
*Guest Editor*

Multi-organ dysfunction is the "normal" condition for many patients admitted to the intensive care unit (ICU). Consequently, the intensivist does not have the luxury of just focusing on the airway and ventilator management, or maintenance of blood pressure, or provision of renal replacement therapy; he/she must be prepared and competent in the diagnosis and management of abnormalities that occur in virtually any organ system. Fortunately, the intensivist does not do this alone—critical care is truly a team sport in the realm of medicine. However, in order to be maximally effective, the intensivist, as the team captain, must have a working knowledge of the possible and likely abnormalities to be encountered in each organ system in order to set the team in the correct direction. In this issue of the *Critical Care Clinics*, we have focused on derangements in the hematologic system that might reasonably be encountered in critically ill patients.

In this issue, the reader will find nine articles written by intensivists or by hematologists, such as myself, with expertise in the hematologic issues frequently encountered, or equally important, considered but not encountered, in ICU patients. In recognizing the importance and frequency of alterations in hemostasis in critically ill patients, five of the articles focus on issues having an impact on the care of patients with hemorrhagic or thrombotic events. Two of the articles address anemia in the ICU. While this is an old problem, our thoughts on the pathophysiology and treatment of the anemic patient have changed, and we believe that these two articles, by reviewing this topic, will provide new insights for our readers and ultimately improve the care of critically ill patients. Last, the discipline of transfusion medicine is also found in this issue in reviews of our current knowledge on transfusion-related acute lung injury and the role of plasmapheresis in critical illness.

Our goal was to produce an issue that the practicing intensivist would use as a reference for the care of his/her patient and also serve as the starting point for

Crit Care Clin 28 (2012) ix–x
http://dx.doi.org/10.1016/j.ccc.2012.04.010
0749-0704/12/$ – see front matter © 2012 Elsevier Inc. All rights reserved.

self-education on a specific topic. I believe that we have succeeded and hope that you will find these reviews to be informative and clinically useful.

Robert I. Parker, MD
Department of Pediatrics
Stony Brook University School of Medicine
Pediatric Hematology/Oncology
Stony Brook Long Island Children's Hospital
HSC T-11, Room 029
100 Nicolls Road
Stony Brook, NY 11794-8111, USA

E-mail address:
Robert.Parker@stonybrookmedicine.edu

# Anemia in the ICU
## Anemia of Chronic Disease Versus Anemia of Acute Illness

Devina Prakash, MBBS

**KEYWORDS**

- Anemia of chronic disease • Anemia of inflammation • Anemia in the ICU • Hepcidin
- Iron deficiency in the ICU • Transfusion and erythropoietin in the ICU

**KEY POINTS**

- Anemia is a common problem in the ICU and is of multifactorial etiology.
- Cytokine mediated increase in Hepcidin is an important mediator of anemia in critically ill patients, leading to poor iron utilization.
- There may be a concurrent iron deficiency in patients with anemia of inflammation which can be difficult to diagnose and treat.
- Transfusing patients with anemia in the ICU to an ideal target hemoglobin is deleterious and restrictive transfusion policies lead to better outcomes.
- Erythropoietin use is associated with worse outcomes and it should be used judiciously.

## EPIDEMIOLOGY

Anemia is a common problem in the intensive care unit (ICU), occurring frequently in critically ill patients. Observational studies indicate an incidence of approximately 95% in patients who have been in the ICU for 3 or more days.[1] The presence of anemia has been associated with worse outcomes including increased lengths of stay and increased mortality.[2] The etiology of anemia is multifactorial and includes the following:

1. Frequent blood sampling; in one study, the average total volume of blood drawn was 41.1 mL per patient during a 24-hour period.[2] The quantity of blood phlebotomized accounted for 49% variation in amount of blood transfused in an observational study by Corwin and colleagues.[3]
2. Clinically apparent or occult blood loss through the gastrointestinal tract.

The author has nothing to disclose.
Division of Pediatric Hematology Oncology, T-11, HSC-2, Room 020, Stony Brook Long Island Children's Hospital, Stony Brook, NY 11794–8111, USA
*E-mail address:* devina.prakash@sbumed.org

Crit Care Clin 28 (2012) 333–343
http://dx.doi.org/10.1016/j.ccc.2012.04.012
0749-0704/12/$ – see front matter © 2012 Elsevier Inc. All rights reserved.

3. Blood loss from preceding trauma.
4. Blood loss as a result of surgical interventions.
5. Impaired production of red cells secondary to a blunted erythropoietin response to anemia in critically ill patients. Erythropoietin (Epo) levels have been found to be inappropriately low in these patients, with a loss of the normal inverse correlation that exists between serum Epo levels and hematocrit levels.[4,5] The blunted Epo response appears to be a result of suppression by inflammatory cytokines.[6] These patients, however, retain their responsiveness to exogenously administered Epo.[7] There is also a direct suppressive effect on erythroid production secondary to direct bone marrow suppression by inflammatory cytokines such as interleukin-1 (IL-1) and tumor necrosis factor-$\alpha$ (TNF-$\alpha$) and inhibitory effects of interferon-$\alpha$, $\beta$, and $\gamma$.
6. It is being increasingly recognized that the anemia in a majority of critically ill patients is a result of poor iron utilization akin to that seen in the so-called anemia of chronic disease. This is now more accurately called anemia of inflammation (AI). Decreased serum iron, serum transferrin, transferrin saturation, and increased ferritin levels have been found in these patients, indicative of an inflammatory profile. In one study of 51 postoperative critically ill patients, decreased serum iron and increased ferritin were found in more than 75% of patients. Forty-one of these patients suffered 56 septic episodes. These were accompanied by a marked decrease in serum transferrin and increase in serum ferritin accompanied by a reduction in hemoglobin ($P<.001$). Recovery from sepsis was accompanied by a significant improvement in hemoglobin, serum iron, and transferrin.[8]

## PATHOPHYSIOLOGY OF ANEMIA OF INFLAMMATION

To understand the pathophsiology of anemia of inflammation, it is important to first understand normal iron metabolism in the body. Iron has the capacity to donate and accept electrons easily, thus interconverting between the ferric ($Fe^{3+}$) and ferrous ($Fe^{2+}$) forms. This makes it a useful component of oxygen binding molecules (hemoglobin and myoglobin), cytochromes, and other enzymes involved in electron transfer reactions. On the flip side, iron must be bound to transporter/storage proteins at all times because free reactive iron causes tissue damage, most likely by catalyzing the production of free oxygen radicals from hydrogen peroxide. For this reason the concentration of iron in biological fluids is tightly regulated. Iron homeostasis in mammals is regulated at the level of intestinal absorption, as the body has no physiologic pathway to increase iron excretion.

A well balanced diet contains about 10 to 20 mg of iron daily, and roughly 10% of dietary iron is absorbed each day (**Fig. 1**). The efficiency of iron absorption can increase up to 20% in response to increased utilization in children secondary to growth, or increased requirements in pregnancy, and with greater iron loss as occurs with menstruation and with minor hemorrhages. A small amount of iron is lost from the body daily, mainly from the shedding of cells containing iron in the gastrointestinal tract and exfoliation of skin cells. About 1 mg of iron is lost per day, though menstruating women lose about 2 mg/day. This is balanced by absorption of 1 to 2 mg iron/day.

Normal adult males have 35 to 45 mg of iron per kilogram of body weight, and total body iron content of 4 to 6 g. Females tend to have lower amounts of body iron secondary to blood loss during menstruation. Roughly 80% of the total iron content is functional, the remainder being in the storage form. Approximately 80% of the functional iron is found bound to hemoglobin; the remainder is contained in myoglobin and iron-containing enzymes such as cytochromes. 20% of iron is stored as either ferritin or hemosiderin.

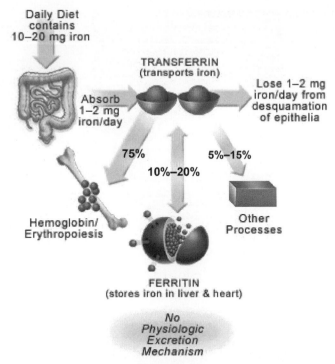

Fig. 1. Normal iron cycle. (*From* Centers for Disease Control. Hemochromatosis (Iron Storage Disease). Available at: http://www.cdc.gov/ncbddd/hemochromatosis/training/index.html.)

The average daily requirement of iron to support erythropoiesis is 20 to 25 mg. However, only a small fraction of this is absorbed from the diet. Most of the daily iron requirement for erythropoiesis is met by recycling of iron from senescent erythrocytes; these are phagocytosed by reticuloendothelial macrophages followed by degradation of hemoglobin. The recycled iron is then made available to the erythroid precursors in the bone marrow.

### Mechanism of Iron Absorption

The absorption of iron and its regulation has become better understood over the last decade (**Fig. 2**). Iron is principally absorbed in the proximal duodenum, where it may be taken up either as ionic iron or as heme iron. Dietary nonheme iron is mainly in the ferric state. It is first reduced to the ferrous state by the enzyme duodenal cytochrome B (DcytB) present at the brush border of the duodenal enterocytes. It then crosses the apical brush border through the transporter divalent metal ion transporter 1 (DMT1). Heme bound iron is transported through a separate pathway, the heme carrier protein (HCP1). Once within the enterocytes, iron has two basic fates depending on iron requirements. If iron requirement is low, the absorbed iron remains sequestered as ferritin and is lost with shedding of the enterocytes. In situations of iron need, iron crosses the basolateral membrane of the enterocyte via the iron export protein ferroportin (FPN). This efflux of iron from the enterocytes is coupled with oxidation from ferrous to ferric iron and is carried out by the heme oxidases hephaestin and ceruloplasmin. **Ferroportin** is the **sole known iron exporter** required for iron efflux

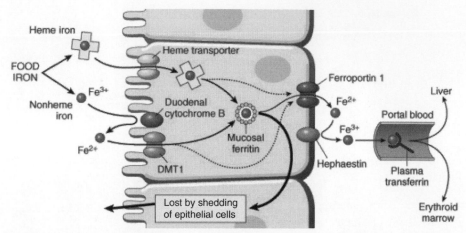

**Fig. 2.** Iron absorption in the duodenum. (*From* Kumar V, Abbas AK, Fausto N, et al. Robbins & Cotran Pathologic Basis of Disease, 8th Edition. Philadelphia: Elsevier, 2009; with permission.)

from all cells that contain iron such as macrophages in the reticuloendothelial system, placental cells that transport iron from mother to fetus, and duodenal enterocytes.[9,10]

### Iron Transport and Storage

The newly absorbed iron is transported in the blood stream bound to the glycoprotein transferrin (TF), which is the principal iron-carrying protein in the systemic circulation. TF has two high-affinity binding sites for iron ($Fe^{3+}$). TF serves three major functions: (1) It allows $Fe^{3+}$ to remain soluble in plasma; (2) it renders iron nontoxic; and (3) it facilitates cellular import of iron by binding to the transferrin receptor (TfR1) on cell surfaces, allowing for endocytosis and release of TF bound iron into the cell where it can be utilized. Transferrin has the ability to bind 330 $\mu$g of iron per deciliter. Normally, about 25% to 45% of transferrin binding sites are filled (measured as percent transferrin saturation). The liver is the main site of storage of absorbed iron. Iron is also found stored in macrophages that recycle iron from senescent red blood cells. Iron is predominantly stored in ferritin molecules. A single ferritin molecule can store up to 4000 iron atoms. A very small amount of iron is found in plasma as ferritin. Serum ferritin averages about 12 to 300 $\mu$g/L. Serum ferritin appears to be in equilibrium with tissue ferritin and is a good reflection of storage iron in normal subjects. It is important to remember, however, that serum ferritin is an acute phase reactant and levels are disproportionately increased in the presence of inflammation, malignancy, and hepatocellular disorders.[11,12]

### Regulation of Iron Homeostasis

Iron homeostasis requires a very tight control on iron absorption in the intestine, closely coupled to body iron requirements. Under normal circumstances, the iron concentration in plasma and extracellular fluid remains in a relatively narrow range despite fluctuating iron supply and demand. Recent discoveries have helped elucidate some of the mechanisms that are required to achieve this, both at a cellular and systemic level.

The major regulators of iron absorption have long been recognized to be body iron stores, bone marrow erythropoietic activity, blood hemoglobin level, hypoxia, and the presence of inflammation.[11]

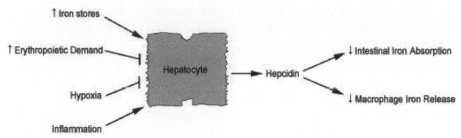

**Fig. 3.** Regulation of hepcidin. (*From* Heeney M, Andrews N. Iron homeostasis and inherited iron overload disorders: an overview. Hematol Oncol Clin of N Am 2004;18(6):1379–403; with permission.)

### Cellular regulation

Intracellular iron levels are detected by two **I**ron **R**egulatory **P**roteins (IRP1/IRP2). The IRPs bind to **I**ron **R**esponsive **E**lements (IRE) located on the mRNA of the protein to be regulated. If the IRE is located on the 3′ region of the mRNA of the protein, binding by the IRP prevents degradation by endonucleases and results in increased stability of the corresponding protein, thus increasing its level. If the IRE is located on the 5′ region, binding by IRP blocks translation and thereby decreases synthesis of the protein.

Thus in low iron states, IRP binding increases stability of transferrin mRNA (reflected as increased TIBC) and decreases synthesis of ferritin mRNA, the converse occurring in high iron states. Other proteins' mRNAs that are regulated by IRPs include DMT1, DcytB, and ferroportin.[11,12] It is not yet understood how the cellular and systemic regulation of iron is coordinated.

### Systemic regulation

Hepcidin, a 25-amino-acid peptide secreted predominantly by hepatocytes, is now recognized to be the **master** regulator of iron homeostasis. It a member of the defensin proteins and is linked to innate immunity.[12] Hepcidin circulates in plasma bound to an $\alpha_2$-macroglobulin and is cleared by the kidney. It is a negative regulator of iron acquisition and its expression is inversely correlated with body iron stores. Hepcidin binds to and induces internalization and degradation of ferroportin, the sole iron export protein found in duodenal enterocytes and macrophages, thus decreasing iron efflux from these cells. Thus iron remains sequestered within these cells. In the duodenal enterocytes, this sequestered iron is shed with sloughing of the cells, resulting in decreased iron absorption by the gut. In the case of the macrophages, iron remains stored in the reticuloendothelial system and cannot be utilized for erythropoiesis.

As the primary target for hepcidin action has been recognized, there has been increasing focus on the mechanism by which hepcidin production is regulated (**Fig. 3**). It is well recognized that hepcidin production is increased in iron sufficiency states but decreased in states of iron deficiency, allowing for greater absorption of iron from the gut. Hepcidin production is also decreased in the presence of hypoxia and under conditions of increased erythropoietic demand, thereby allowing for increased iron delivery to the bone marrow erythroid progenitors.

Dysregulation of hepcidin synthesis can occur in conditions characterized by ineffective erythropoiesis (intramedullary hemolysis) such as that present in thalassemia intermedia syndromes. This results in decreased hepcidin levels and accounts for the disproportionately increased iron absorption and resulting iron overload seen in this condition. Another example is the increased hepcidin synthesis that occurs in the presence of infections and inflammatory disorders. The increased hepcidin synthesis is cytokine mediated (predominantly IL-6) and contributes to the development of anemia of inflammation characterized by hypoferremia and anemia despite adequate iron stores.

### Genes Involved in Regulation of Hepcidin

Increasing understanding of the pathogenesis of inherited disorders of iron metabolism has contributed greatly to increased understanding of iron homeostasis. Mutations in a number of genes, including hemojuvelin (HJV), HFE, and transferrin receptor 2 (TfR2), lead to iron overloading and hemochromatosis. This mimics the iron loading seen with hepcidin gene mutations that result in hepcidin deficiency. It has now been established that HJV, HFE, and TfR2 are all parts of the same regulatory pathway. TfR2 appears to act as an iron sensing protein. The bone morphogenetic protein (BMP)–SMAD pathway appears to be central to the final regulation of hepcidin and is closely linked to HJV, HFE, and TfR2.[11–13]

There has been much interest in identifying the mechanism by which increased erythropoietic activity regulates hepcidin synthesis. The regulation of hepcidin by erythropoietic activity is now thought to be mediated by the recently described growth differentiation factor 15 (GDF15). Levels of GDF15 are elevated in patients with thalassemia intermedia. GDF-15 suppresses synthesis of hepcidin and allows for increased iron absorption regardless of iron body stores. A newly described hypoxia inducible factor (HIF) has also been found to suppress hepcidin synthesis in hypoxic mice and may be the pathway of increased iron absorption seen in conditions of hypoxia.[11,13]

### ANEMIA OF INFLAMMATION

Anemia of Inflammation (AI) is now the preferred name for the anemia of chronic disease as it develops acutely in states of inflammation. It is the second most common cause of anemia after iron deficiency. Inflammation causes a mild to moderate normocytic, normochromic anemia associated with abnormal iron utilization. The hallmark of the disorder is a decrease in serum iron and transferrin saturation in the presence of elevated ferritin.[14] These findings point to inhibition of iron recycling by macrophages, typically seen in hepcidin excess.

Hepcidin is induced by inflammation resulting in the classic anemia of inflammation characterized by hypoferremia in the presence of increase iron stores. Iron is essential for bacterial growth and the sequestration of iron in inflammation appears to be a defense mechanism by vertebrates to starve infecting bacteria iron. As stated earlier, IL-6 is the most important inducer of hepcidin. In human volunteers, infusion of IL-6 results in a five- to sevenfold increase in urinary hepcidin levels within 2 hours of infusion.[12,15] This is accompanied by a 30% decrease in serum iron and transferrin saturation within hours of the infusion. In addition to hepatocyte synthesis of hepcidin, several studies have demonstrated hepcidin production by macrophages exposed to bacterial stimulation. This may allow for degradation of macrophage ferroportin and decreased availability of iron locally to bacterial.[16] Immune-mediated depression of erythropoiesis in conjunction with reduced erythropoietin production further exacerbates the anemia.

### ANEMIA OF INFLAMMATION WITH CONCURRENT IRON DEFICIENCY

Critically ill patients loose large amounts of blood for various reasons such as phlebotomy, surgical procedures, and occult gastrointestinal blood loss.[2,3,17] It has

**Table 1**
**Indices to differentiate ID, AI, and concurrent AI/IDA**

| | ID | AI | AI/IDA |
|---|---|---|---|
| Iron | ↓ ↓ | ↓ ↓ | ↓ ↓ |
| Transferrin | ↑ ↑ | ↓ ↓ | N or ↓ |
| Transferrin sat. | ↓ ↓ | ↓ ↓ | ↓ ↓ |
| Ferritin | ↓ ↓ | ↑ ↑ | N or ↑ |
| Zinc protoporphyrin | ↑ ↑ | N or ↑ | ↑ ↑ |
| sTfR | ↑ ↑ | ↓ ↓ | ↑ |
| sTfR/log ferritin | ↑ ↑ | ↓ | ↑ |
| Hepcidin | ↓ ↓ | ↑ ↑ | N or ↓ |
| C-reactive protein | N | ↑ ↑ | ↑ |

*Data from* Heming N, Montravers P, Lasocki S. Iron deficiency in critically ill patients: highlighting the role of hepcidin. Crit Care 2011;15:210–6.
*Abbreviations:* N, normal; ↑, increased; ↓, decreased.

been estimated that this may amount to a median iron loss of as much as 64 mg/day.[17] Because the daily absorption of iron is only 1-2 mg, this is very likely to lead to iron deficiency. Thus, there are two competing effects on iron metabolism in the presence of coexisting inflammation and iron deficiency. Inflammation was thought to be the predominant contributor to anemia in the ICU but recent studies indicate that iron deficiency may be equally if not more important. Iron deficiency may occur in up to 40% of very ill patients.[18] Diagnosis of iron-deficiency anemia (IDA) in patients with AI is challenging (**Table 1**). In the presence of inflammation, the usual parameters used to diagnose iron deficiency are no longer valid. Serum iron and transferrin saturation are reduced. Serum ferritin levels are elevated and no longer indicative of iron deficiency. It is important to make the diagnosis of IDA as these patients would benefit from iron supplementation, whereas iron supplementation in patients with AI could be deleterious, because of the ability of iron to promote bacterial growth and cause oxidative tissue damage. Various indices have been studied to help discriminate between the two conditions. These include red cell zinc protoporphyrin, soluble transferrin receptors (sTfR), and sTfR/log ferritin ratios.[18–20]

It was postulated that hepcidin levels may be useful as a marker of IDA in the presence of AI since hepcidin is the master regulator of iron homeostasis. Levels of hepcidin are markedly reduced in the presence of IDA; conversely, they are elevated in AI. A prospective observational study was performed by Lasocki and colleagues to determine the cutoff value and diagnostic accuracy of hepcidin levels to diagnose IDA in the presence of AI.[19] A total of 128 iron profiles were analyzed in 51 patients. Median hepcidin levels were 80.5 $\mu$g/L in IDA and 526.6 $\mu$g/L in patients with AI. Hepcidin levels declined progressively in eight patients who developed iron deficiency. A threshold level of 129.5 $\mu$g/L of hepcidin permitted a diagnosis of iron deficiency. The authors demonstrated that hepcidin levels decline with iron deficiency even in the presence of inflammation. This finding has been confirmed in other studies.[20] Hepcidin assays are not available to clinicians at this time. These results also require validation in larger clinical studies.

## TREATMENT OPTIONS

The rationale for treatment of AI is twofold: (1) to improve oxygen delivery to tissues and (2) because of the poorer prognosis associated with its presence.

Therapy for anemia in the ICU has traditionally leaned toward correcting the hemoglobin to an arbitrary "normal" because of the perceived risk of anemia-associated morbidity and mortality. There has been a sea change over the last decade in the management of anemia in the face of better understanding of the pathophysiology of anemia.

### Red Cell Transfusions

Blood transfusions have been used in critically ill anemic patients with the intent of improving oxygen delivery to tissues. More than 50% of patients admitted to the ICU receive blood transfusions.[3] This number increases to 85% in those with longer length of stay (>7 days).[3]

A target hemoglobin of 10 g/dL has been accepted as a minimum threshold to transfuse since its first proposal in 1942: the 10/30 rule.[21] This practice remained unchanged for decades despite the lack of evidence to support its use. With increasing recognition of risks associated with blood transfusions such as transmission of infections, TRALI, allergic reactions, fluid overload, and immunomodulation, there has been a more critical appraisal of the need of blood transfusions in this population of patients. Two large observational studies defined the use of blood transfusions in the ICU. The first included 1136 patients from 145 western European ICUs.[2] The transfusion rate during the ICU stay was 37%. Mortality rates were significantly higher in patients who were transfused versus those who were not. There was a dose–response effect with a higher mortality seen in patients receiving increased number of transfusions. The second study, the CRIT study showed that the number of red cell transfusions a patient received in the ICU was independently associated with increased mortality.[22] In 90% of patients, low hemoglobin was noted as one of the indications for transfusion, indicating that arbitrary triggers still dictate transfusion practice A multicenter, randomized, controlled trial comparing restricted (transfusion for hemoglobin <7g/dL to maintain target hemoglobin of 7–9.0 g/dL) with liberal transfusions (transfusion for hemoglobin <10 g/dL to maintain target hemoglobin 10–12 g/dL) in critically ill patients carried out by the Transfusion Requirements in Critical Care Investigations (TRICC) showed that a restrictive strategy is at least as good as the more liberal one and significantly better in patients who were less acutely ill and younger than 55 years. The only exceptions were patients with acute myocardial ischemia.[23] Of interest, red blood transfusions do not appear to increase oxygen consumption ($\dot{V}o_2$) by tissues even though oxygen delivery ($Do_2$) increases significantly.[24,25]

A significant association has been found between the number of red blood cell units transfused and subsequent development of infections in patients after trauma and in postoperative patients. Similar associations have been found between red blood transfusions and development of nosocomial infections in critically sick patients. This is thought to be a result of immunomodulation induced by transfused allogeneic blood (transfusion related immunomodulation or TRIM). The mechanism of TRIM is not clearly understood. Allogeneic white blood cells (WBCs) have been considered a cause.[26] Studies looking at the effect of leukoreduction on reducing infections are contradictory and no clear consensus has been reached.[27] Further discussion on this issue is beyond the scope of this article.

Current recommendations advocate the use of restricted red blood cell transfusion practice, limiting transfusions to those clinically indicated rather than transfusing to an "ideal" target hematocrit.

## Erythropoietic Agents

Erythropoietic agents have been used in critically ill patients to attempt to decrease the need for blood transfusions. The demonstration of a relative deficiency of Epo for degree of anemia[4] led to the interest in using Epo as a therapeutic agent. Early studies focused on looking for evidence of bone marrow response to exogenous Epo as evidenced by increase in reticulocyte count and serum transferrin receptor but did not evaluate effect on clinical outcomes.[7] Corwin and colleagues performed a prospective, randomized, placebo-controlled trial in which they enrolled 1460 patients.[28] There was no reduction in the number of patients who required a transfusion or in the number of transfusions received in the treated as compared to the the placebo group. Use of Epo was associated with a significant increase in the incidence of thrombosis. Mortality rates were lower in the Epo group, especially in a subgroup of patients with trauma who were in the ICU for more than 48 hours. The etiology of reduced mortality was unclear. However, it did not appear to be related to reduction in use of blood products. The authors hypothesize that this may be the result of the non-erythropoietic effects of Epo, that is, its antiapoptotic effect and tissue protective effects in the face of ischemia and hypoxia.[29] A meta-analysis of nine randomized, controlled trials involving critically ill patients receiving Epo, did not find any difference in overall mortality, length of stay or in the duration of mechanical ventilation. The reduction in transfusion requirement was 0.41 units per patient in the Epo group.[30] There does not appear to be any clear benefit in the use of Epo to ameliorate anemia in critically ill patients. In view of the increased risk of thrombosis and other described risks such as increased risk of cancer recurrence, it should be used only in the confines of a clinical trial.

## Iron Therapy

The recognition of a significant subgroup of critically ill patients with both AI and IDA suggests a possible role for iron therapy. The difficulty lies in accurate diagnosis because the tests with the best discriminatory power such as sTfR/log ferritin ratios and hepcidin levels are not commercially available and have not been clinically validated.[19,20] It also must be kept in mind that iron can cause oxidative stress and theoretically increase the risk of bacterial infection. However, observational studies have not shown any association between iron administration and risk for infection.[31]

Iron may be administered orally or intravenously. It is important to remember that absorption of oral iron may be reduced in patients with AI because of the effect of hepcidin mediated reduction of ferroportin in duodenal enterocytes. Interestingly, the study by Pieracci using oral iron (325 mg $FeSO_4$ 3 times/day) in critically ill patients documented a decrease in transfusion requirements and no increase in incidence of infections.[31,32] Iron supplementation should be used in patients who are on erythropoietic agents for optimal response. Iron therapy is not recommended for patients with AI who have a high ferritin level and no suspicion of concurrent iron deficiency.[19]

An algorithm has been suggested by Heming and colleagues[18] for diagnosis and treatment of IDA and IA, though it has not been clinically validated. The authors propose the use of C-reactive protein (CRP), serum ferritin, sTfR/log ferritin ratios, and hepcidin levels to make a decision regarding use of iron. Patients are considered to have both IDA and AI if they have reduced hepcidin levels and reduced sTfR/log ferritin ratios in the face of elevated CRP and ferritin levels. These patients would likely benefit from judicious administration of iron.

### Novel Therapies

A better understanding of the role played by hepcidin in iron regulation and development of AI has opened the door to development of new therapies targeting this pathway. Hepcidin antagonists are expected to be useful in states of hepcidin excess as is seen in AI.

Hepcidin depletion by neutralizing antibodies or by hepcidin small interfering RNAs (siRNAs) in conjunction with Epo corrected anemia in a mouse model of AI.[33] In human patients with Castleman disease, a lymphoproliferative disorder associated with elevated IL-6 levels, administration of anti-IL-6 antibodies reduces serum hepcidin levels.[34] Hepcidin levels may also be altered by targeting bone morphogenetic protein (BMP) pathway, which is essential in regulation of hepcidin using a BMP receptor inhibitor dorsomorphin.[35] Other possible targets to reduce hepcidin effect include inhibition of binding with ferroportin.[12]

### REFERENCES

1. Corwin HL, Rodriguez RM, Pearl RG, et al. Erythropoietin response in critically ill patients. Crit Care Med 1997;25(Suppl 1):82.
2. Vincent JL, Baron JF, Reinhart K, et al. Anemia and blood transfusions in critically ill patients. JAMA 2002;288:1499–507.
3. Corwin H, Parsonnet KC, Gettinger A. RBC transfusion in the ICU: is there a reason? Chest 1995;108:767–71.
4. Rogiers P, Zhang H, Leeman M, et al. Erythropoietin response is blunted in critically ill patients. Intensive Care Med 1997;23:159–62.
5. Eliot JM, Virankabutra T, Jones S, et al. Erythropoietin mimics the acute phase response in critical illness. Crit Care 2003;7:R35–40.
6. Jelkmann W. Proinflammatory cytokines lowering erythropoietin production. J Interferon Cytokine Res 1998;18:555–9.
7. van Iperan CE, Gaillard CAJM, Kraaijenhagen RJ, et al. Response of erythropoiesis and iron metabolism to recombinant human erythropoietin in intensive care unit patients. Crit Care Med 2000;28:2773–8.
8. Bobbio-Pallavicini F, Verde G, Spriano P, et al. Body iron status in critically ill patients: significance of serum ferritin. Intensive Care Med 1989;15:171–8.
9. Fleming RE. Advances in understanding the molecular basis for the regulation of dietary iron absorption. Curr Opin Gastroenterol 2005;21:201–6.
10. Anderson GJ, Frazer DM, Mclaren GD. Iron absorption and metabolism. Curr Opin Gastroenterol 2009;25:129–35.
11. Nemeth E. Iron regulation and erythropoiesis. Curr Opin Hematol 2008;15:169–75.
12. Hentze MW, Muckenthaler MU, Galy B, et al. Two to tango: regulation of mammalian iron metabolism. Cell 2010;142:24–38.
13. Andrews NC. Disorders of iron metabolism. N Engl J Med 1999;341:1986–95.
14. Wiess G, Goodnough LT. Anemia of chronic disease. N Engl J Med 2005;352:1011–23.
15. Nemeth E, Ganz T. Regulation of iron metabolism by hepcidin. Ann Rev Nutr 2006;26:323–42.
16. Peyssonnaux C, Zinkermagel AS, Datta V, et al. TLR4-dependent hepcidin expression by myeloid cells in response to bacterial patogens. Blood 2006;107:3727–32.

17. von Ahsen N, Muller C, Serke S, et al. Important role of nondiagnostic blood loss and blunted erythropoietic response in the anemia of medical intensive care patients. Crit Care Med 1999;27:2630–9.
18. Heming N, Montravers P, Lasocki S. Iron deficiency in critically ill patients: highlighting the role of hepcidin. Crit Care 2011;15:210–6.
19. Lasocki S, Baron G, Driss F. Diagnostic accuracy of serum hepcidin for iron deficiency in critically ill patients with anemia. Intensive Care Med 2010;36:1044–8.
20. Theurl I, Aigner E, Theuri M, et al. Regulation of iron homeostasis in anemia of chronic disease and iron deficiency anemia: diagnostic and therapeutic implications. Blood 2009;113:5277–86.
21. Adam RC, Lundy JS. Anesthesia in cases of poor risk: some suggestions for reducing the risk. Surg Gynecol Obstet 1942;74:1011–101.
22. Corwin H, Gettinger A, Pearl RG, et al. The CRIT study: anemia and blood transfusions in the critically ill—current practice in the United States. Crit Care Med 2004;32:39–52.
23. Hebert PC, Wells G, Blajchman A. A multicenter, randomized, controlled clinical trial of transfusion requirements in critical care. N Engl J Med 1999;340:409–17.
24. Conrad SA, Dietrich KA, Hebert CA, et al. Effect of red cell transfusion on oxygen consumption following fluid resuscitation in septic shock. Circ Shock 1990;31:419–29.
25. Shah DM, Gottlieb ME, Rahm RL, et al. Failure of red blood cell transfusion to increase oxygen transport or mixed venous $Po_2$ in injured patients. J Trauma 1982;22:741–6.
26. Vamvakas EC, Blajchman MA. Deleterious clinical effects of transfusion-associated immunomodulation: fact or fiction? Blood 2001;97:1180–95.
27. Dzik WH, Anderson JK, O'Neil EM, et al. A prospective, randomized clinical trial of universal WBC reduction. Transfusion 2002;42:1114–22.
28. Corwin H, Gettinger A, Fabian T, et al. Efficacy and safety of epoietin alfa in critically ill patients. N Engl J Med 2007;357:965–76.
29. Coleman T, Brines M. Science review: recombinant human erythropoietin in critical illness: a role beyond anemia? Crit Care 2004;8:337–41.
30. Zarychanski R, Turgeon AF, McIntyre L. Erythropoietin-receptor agonists in critically ill patients: a meta-analysis of randomized controlled trials. CMAJ 2007;177:725–34.
31. Hoen B, Paul-Dauphin A, Kessler M. Intravenous iron administration does not significantly increase the risk of bacteremia in chronic hemodialyis patients. Clin Nephrol 2002;57:457–61.
32. Pieracci FM, Henderson P, Rodney JR, et al. Randomized, double blind, placebo controlled trial of effects of enteral iron supplementation on anemia and risk of infection during surgical clinical illness. Surg Infect 2009;10:9–19.
33. Sasu BJ, Cooke KS, Arvedson TL, et al. Anti hepcidin antibody treatment modulates iron metabolism and is effective in a mouse model of inflammation induced anemia. Blood 2010;115:3616–24.
34. Song SJ, Tomosugi N, Kawabata H, et al. Downregulation of hepcidin resulting from long term treatment with an anti IL-6 receptor antibody (tocilizumab) improves anemia of inflammation in multicentric Castleman's disease. Blood 2010;116:3627–34.
35. Yu PB, Hong CC, Sachidanandan C, et al. Dorsomorphin inhibits BMP signal required for embryogenesis and iron metabolism. Nat Chem Biol 2008;4:33–41.

# The Use of Erythropoiesis-Stimulating Agents in the Intensive Care Unit

Michael Piagnerelli, MD, PhD[a], Jean-Louis Vincent, MD, PhD[b],*

## KEYWORDS

- Iron • Erythropoietin • Anemia • Transfusion

## KEY POINTS

- Erythropoietin (EPO) regulates red blood cell (RBC) production in the bone marrow. In critically ill patients, the normal EPO response to anemia seems to be blunted and this effect may contribute to the anemia in these patients.
- Limiting the occurrence and severity of anemia by using erythropoietic agents (iron and/or recombinant EPO) could be an attractive management strategy in critically ill patients.
- Iron can stimulate erythropoiesis, but more information regarding optimal dosing, route of administration, and potential side effects (increased infections) are needed before it can be routinely used.
- Randomized controlled trials of EPO use in critically ill patients have generated conflicting results. The largest study in a heterogeneous group of anemic ICU patients found no decrease in RBC transfusions and no effect on mortality rates, except perhaps in patients with trauma; this study also reported increased thrombotic events with EPO.
- EPO has various pleiotropic effects (anti-apoptosis, angiogenesis) and may be better targeted at specific subgroups of anemic ICU patients (for example, those with brain trauma).

## INTRODUCTION

Anemia, as defined by the World Health Organization,[1] is common in the general population. In a study on the nutritional habits of approximately 40,000 noninstitutionalized individuals, the prevalence of anemia was reported to be 12% in females of

Conflicts of interest: The authors declare they have no conflicts of interest related to this article.
[a] Department of Intensive Care, CHU-Charleroi, Boulevard Zoé Drion 1, Université Libre de Bruxelles, 6000-Charleroi, Belgium; [b] Department of Intensive Care, Erasme Hospital, Université Libre de Bruxelles, Route de Lennik, 808, 1070-Brussels, Belgium
* Corresponding author.
E-mail address: jlvincent@ulb.ac.be

reproductive age, 16% in men aged 75 to 84, and as high as 20% in men older than 85.[2] Anemia is much more common in critically ill patients treated in an intensive care unit (ICU). In the European Anemia and Blood Transfusion in Critical Care study, 63% of the 3534 critically ill patients included had a hemoglobin level less than 12 g/dL, and in 29% it was below 10 g/dL.[3] A prospective observational study in the United States reported similar results.[4] In a multiinstitution Scottish study, anemia was even more common, with 55% of the 174 patients studied having a hemoglobin level less than 9 g/dL.[5]

The presence of anemia at ICU admission could be a marker of the severity of disease. In 1988, Carson and colleagues[6] showed, in surgical patients who declined a red blood cell (RBC) transfusion for religious reasons, that there was a significant association between the severity of preoperative anemia and 30-day mortality; the mortality was 7.1% for nonanemic patients (hemoglobin ≥10 g/dL) and increased to 62% in patients with a hemoglobin concentration less than 6 g/dL. Mudumbai and colleagues[7] recently reported increased long-term mortality in critically ill patients admitted to the ICU with a hematocrit less than 25% and who were not transfused during their ICU stay. Anemia present during an ICU stay is often still present 6 months after ICU discharge. In a small study, Bateman and colleagues[8] observed a persistent low hematocrit with low reticulocyte count suggesting decreased RBC production in the bone marrow, and a blunted erythropoietin response to anemia at 6 months in 50% of patients discharged from the ICU with a hemoglobin level under 10 g/dL.

The severity of anemia increases during the ICU stay[9] and often requires RBC transfusion.[10] More than 70% of patients with an ICU length of stay over 1 week may receive an RBC transfusion.[11] In a study examining ICU transfusion practice and mortality, a third of all ICU admissions received a RBC transfusion,[12] although transfusion policies have become more restrictive[13–17] in recent years with increased awareness of the possible side effects of this intervention, including bacteria, virus or prion transmission, transfusion-related immunomodulation, transfusion-associated circulatory overload, and transfusion-related acute lung injury.

To limit RBC transfusions in ICU patients, erythropoietic stimulating agents could be used to stimulate the bone marrow. To use these agents, we need to understand the pathophysiology of anemia in critically ill patients. Two erythropoietic agents could potentially be administered, together or separately: iron and erythropoietin (EPO). In this article the authors review iron and EPO metabolism and the literature regarding their administration in critically ill patients.

## IRON

Anemia in the critically ill patient is a multifactorial phenomenon and is the result not only of blood losses, but also of an inflammatory response with blunted EPO production, abnormalities in iron metabolism, and altered proliferation and differentiation of marrow erythroid precursors.[18]

Alterations in iron metabolism play a central role in the development of anemia. Most of the body's iron content (4–5 g) is incorporated into hemoglobin (2.5 g) in developing erythroid precursors and mature RBCs, but this process is rapidly altered with the acute phase reaction. Indeed, in just a few hours, proinflammatory and antiinflammatory cytokines cause a decrease in blood iron levels, called functional iron deficiency. Hepcidin, a peptide synthesized by the liver and the macrophages, which decreases ferroportin expression on macrophages and enterocytes to limit the availability of free serum iron, is rapidly released in greater amounts (**Fig. 1**).[19–21] Hepcidin is now considered to be the key mediator of inflammation-induced anemia.

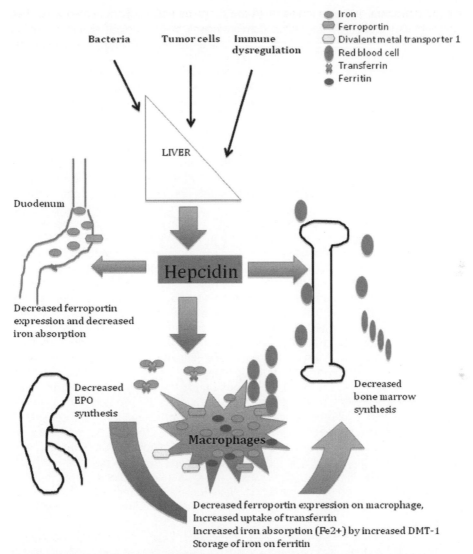

**Fig. 1.** Role of hepcidin in the pathophysiology of anemia in critically ill patients. Hepcidin produced by the liver is the key protein of iron metabolism, which inhibits duodenal absorption of iron by decreased expression of ferroportin. Macrophages increase the expression of the divalent metal transporter 1 (DMT1) due to stimulation by inflammatory cytokines and stimulate the uptake of iron. IL-10 (an antiinflammatory cytokine) upregulates transferrin receptor expression and increases transferrin-receptor-mediated uptake of transferrin-bound iron into monocytes. In addition, activated macrophages phagocytose and degrade senescent erythrocytes for the recycling of iron. Moreover, hepcidin decreases the expression of ferroportin on the macrophage surface, and thus inhibits iron export from macrophages.

Proinflammatory cytokines, such as tumor necrosis factor (TNF)-$\alpha$, interleukin (IL)-1$\beta$, and IL-6, induce the transcription and the translation of ferritin (the protein responsible for iron storage). Intracellular iron content modulates the binding affinity of cytoplasmic iron regulatory proteins (IRP)-1 and IRP-2, with iron-responsive elements, and rapidly decreases the messenger RNA (mRNA) expression of transferrin receptors inducing a decrease in transferrin concentrations (the principal iron-transporting glycoprotein).[22,23] All these modifications result in decreased serum iron concentrations (see **Fig. 1**).

Several studies have reported alterations in iron status in nonbleeding ICU patients (post surgery, trauma, or medical, with or without sepsis).[24–26] The results from most of these studies have been summarized elsewhere.[27] All of them had limitations preventing the extrapolation of their conclusions to ICU patients. First, several reported only single measurements of iron metabolism.[24,25] Second, the time delay between the observed alterations in iron status and the onset of inflammation was not well-defined.[25,28] Third, several studies included patients with comorbidities that can alter iron metabolism, including chronic renal failure, cirrhosis, and hematologic diseases with low or high RBC mean corpuscular volume.[24,26] Finally, patients who had recently received a blood transfusion were not always excluded[24,26] despite the iron load provided by RBC transfusions.[29,30] For these reasons, Piagnerelli and colleagues investigated the time course of iron metabolism in selected critically ill patients with and without sepsis.[31] They only included patients with a short delay between hospital and ICU admission to minimize alterations of iron metabolism occurring because of a prolonged inflammatory process. They also excluded patients with cirrhosis or hematologic diseases and those who were transfused during their ICU stay. The authors observed alterations in iron metabolism already at ICU admission (increased ferritin, decreased iron, transferrin, and transferrin saturation) for septic patients, with lower reticulocyte counts and EPO concentrations, despite being anemic. More interesting, the nonseptic patients had the same degree of alterations, but these abnormalities developed later during their ICU admission (at day 3). These alterations persisted in both groups during the 5-day study period.[31] With this study, the authors confirmed the rapid alteration of iron metabolism in septic patients, but the real take-home message is that they observed the same severity of alterations in nonseptic patients with less inflammation. Because reticulocyte production by the bone marrow is influenced by the inflammatory status (TNF, IL-1, and IL-6), these nonseptic critically ill patients may perhaps be more responsive to iron supplementation to stimulate erythropoiesis. This particular population is perhaps the ideal population for iron supplementation. Nevertheless, this suggestion needs to be confirmed by randomized controlled trials (RCTs) comparing iron supplementation and placebo.

Before starting such a study, a real consensus about the criteria for iron deficiency in patients with inflammation is needed. Indeed, several criteria can be found in the literature including ferritin less than 100 mcg/L,[24] transferrin saturation under 15%,[32] erythrocyte zinc protoporphyrin over 1.24 $\mu$mol/L RBC,[33] hypochromic RBCs greater than 10%,[25] hemoglobin reticulocyte content under 29 pg,[34] or the concentration of transferrin receptors divided by the log of ferritin above 2.[23] Measurements of hepcidin may represent a future method of diagnosing iron deficiency during inflammation, but rapid measurements and clear cutoff values are not yet available in critically ill patients.[35]

Iron administration could be an attractive way to limit the development of anemia in critically ill patients but has not really been tried because of possible unwanted effects:

1. Iron concentrations remain very low during inflammatory states, as commonly observed in critically ill patients.[31] For this reason, optimal supplementation doses to stimulate erythropoiesis without adverse effects have not been determined.

Increasing the effective iron concentration to the bone marrow could be difficult and may need large amounts of iron. In inflammatory states, hepcidin concentrations increase first, and rapidly already within a few hours,[19] and this increases iron storage in the macrophages and inhibits duodenal iron absorption (see **Fig. 1**). Increased ferritin concentrations also limit iron mobilization. Because of these changes in the iron protein, administered iron may perhaps be rapidly stored without any physiologic efficacy, especially on the bone marrow. Some recent data may lead this hypothesis to be revisited. Hepcidin levels were lower than expected in critically ill patients despite an inflammatory process.[35] Before this study in critically ill patients, Lasocki and colleagues[36] tried to reproduce in an animal model of sepsis the pathophysiology of anemia due to repeated phlebotomies, as observed in septic critically ill patients. For this purpose, these investigators compared hepcidin concentrations in several groups of animals: anemic mice with sepsis induced by intraperitoneal injection of lipopolysaccharide associated with zymosan injection after 1 week, septic animals with stimulated erythropoiesis induced by repeated phlebotomy or by EPO, anemic mice treated with EPO, and anemic mice due to repeated phlebotomy. These investigators showed that mice with stimulated erythropoiesis had downregulated liver hepcidin mRNA, independently of the presence of sepsis, and a high liver expression of IL-6. These investigators also looked at the iron store in the spleen and the expression of ferroportin in liver Kupffer cells. They observed decreased ferroportin expression and presence of iron deposits on spleen macrophages in septic animals compared with the other groups. When septic animals became anemic as a result of phlebotomy or EPO, the spleen iron content decreased. With this model of anemic septic mice with stimulated erythropoiesis, the investigators concluded that erythropoiesis stimulation predominates over inflammation for hepcidin regulation and is associated with macrophage iron mobilization.[36]

Confirming the role of stimulated erythropoiesis as a trigger of iron mobilization, Theurl and colleagues[21] observed, in rats with anemia of chronic disease, a persistence of duodenal iron absorption only in animals with stimulated erythropoiesis. All of these studies suggest a possible mobilization of the iron store despite inflammation and synthesis of hepcidin.

2. Iron may participate in the production and/or the persistence of inflammation by synthesis of reactive oxygen species. Indeed, according to the Fenton reaction, iron can react with hydrogen peroxide to generate hydroxyl radicals:

$$Fe^{2+} + H_2O_2 ----> Fe^{3+} + .OH + OH^-$$
$$Fe^{3+} + H_2O_2 ----> Fe^{2+} + .OOH + H^+$$

This circulating nontransferrin bound iron (free iron) could induce tissue damage and initiates local inflammation as observed by Hod and colleagues[30] in a mouse model.

3. Iron administration may promote infections. In an animal model of peritonitis, Javadi and colleagues[37] observed significantly increased mortality rates in animals treated with iron. These results should be analyzed with caution, however, because these animals received very high doses of iron (daily subcutaneous dose of 5 mg/mL with a total of five doses) and were not iron-deficient at baseline. In human volunteers, Hod and colleagues[38] reported an increase in nontransferrin bound iron and transferrin saturation only after transfusion of old stored RBCs (40–42 days) compared with "fresh" RBCs (3–7 days). Indeed, as reported by others,[29] free iron in the RBC units increased in relation to the length of storage. In vitro incubation with *Escherichia coli* of serum from patients transfused with older RBCs

favored bacterial proliferation, confirming the deleterious role of iron on infection.[38] However, although Brasseur and colleagues also observed increased iron levels after transfusions of stored RBCs (>21 days) in critically ill patients, these alterations were not associated with any oxidative stress.[39] On the other hand, iron depletion could have some immunosuppressive effects by decreasing the oxidative burst and phagocytosis of the neutrophils,[40] and correction of this depletion could ameliorate the immune status.

If iron is administered to ICU patients, the intravenous route seems preferable because of the possible effects of hepcidin on duodenal iron absorption and the adverse effects of oral iron administration (ileus). Nevertheless, few data are available concerning iron supplementation in critically ill patients. For example, van Iperen and colleagues[41] did not observe significant modifications in reticulocyte count after intravenous injection of low doses of iron (20 mg/d for 3 weeks) compared with iron with EPO. A limitation of this study is the very low dose of iron administered. In a multicenter study, Vincent and colleagues[42] compared the effects of iron (150 mg/d orally) with EPO and iron in 73 anemic ICU patients. There were no significant differences in reticulocyte or hemoglobin concentrations during the study, but the area under the curve for reticulocytes was greater for EPO and iron compared with iron alone, suggesting that the degree of erythropoiesis in critically ill patients was primarily related to the total dose of EPO administered.[42]

In contrast, in a randomized, double-bind, placebo-controlled trial, Pieracci and colleagues[43] observed a significant reduction in RBC transfusions (30 vs 45%) in 97 anemic surgical patients treated with oral ferrous sulfate 325 mg three times a day. There were no differences in the incidence of infections (47 vs 49%), antibiotic days, lengths of ICU stay, or mortality rates (9.4% vs 9.9%; $P = .62$) between groups. This study with iron supplementation as the only erythropoietic agent used, compared with placebo, is the first controlled trial realized in critically ill patients. The results of this study are very exciting but need confirmation in larger multicenter randomized trials.

In conclusion, iron metabolism is very complex and rapidly altered in critically ill patients. Low iron concentrations contribute to the anemia of critically ill patients. Few data are available on the time course of iron concentrations in ICU patients or on the effects of iron supplementation. Consensus on definitions of iron deficiency using a marker of iron dysfunction (eg, hepcidin) is needed before iron administration can really be assessed in ICU patients. The appropriate dose to limit the risk of side effects, including the production of reactive oxygen species or increased infection, must also be established. For these reasons, studies assessing the time course of hepcidin in critically ill patients with and without sepsis and the relationship between hepcidin concentrations and inflammation (for example, the hepcidin/C-reactive protein ratio) are initially needed. Indeed, hepcidin is an interesting marker of duodenal iron absorption and iron mobilization. RCTs comparing several doses of iron supplementation in patients with low inflammatory syndromes, such as nonseptic critically ill patients, are then needed to determine the optimal dose to prevent anemia in critically ill patients, but also to avoid deleterious effects.

## ERYTHROPOIETIN

EPO is a 30.4 kDa glycoprotein produced by the kidney, known mostly for its physiologic function in regulating RBC production in the bone marrow. The normal EPO response to anemia seems to be blunted in critically ill patients with or without renal failure, so that inadequate EPO production may contribute to anemia in these patients.[44] Nevertheless, as observed by Elliot and colleagues[45] and

Vialet and colleagues,[46] EPO concentrations may mimic those of acute phase proteins with increased concentrations at ICU admission and decreased levels after several days. Indeed, Elliot and colleagues[45] observed significantly higher EPO concentrations during the first 3 days of ICU admission in 25 critically ill patients with acute renal failure compared with those without. After 3 days, EPO levels decreased and were identical to those of nonhospitalized anemic patients despite higher IL-6 concentrations.

Although erythropoiesis is limited in critically ill patients because of inflammatory mediators, functional iron deficiency, and blunted EPO concentrations in relation to the degree of anemia, the bone marrow of these patients seems to be able to respond to the administration of exogenous EPO as evidenced by significant increases in reticulocyte counts and serum transferrin receptor concentrations.[41] Indeed, EPO favors the transformation of late burst-forming units to colony-forming units and finally erythroblasts and reticulocytes. This erythroid differentiation was studied by Claessens and colleagues[47] in patients with septic shock who developed early onset of anemia (hemoglobin concentrations <10 g/dL in the first 48 hours of ICU admission). These investigators observed increased apoptosis of glycophorin A (the most important RBC membrane protein)-erythroid precursors in the bone marrow of these patients, suggesting a blocking effect on the differentiation of the erythroid progenitor cells. Interestingly, these investigators observed that in vitro incubation with high doses of recombinant EPO could restore this differentiation process[47] and permit the formation of erythroblasts.

All these arguments support administration of recombinant EPO as an erythropoietic agent in critically ill patients to limit the development of anemia and avoid RBC transfusions. In addition to its erythropoietic effects, EPO may also have beneficial roles related to its properties against apoptosis. The authors identified 13 studies of EPO administration in critically ill patients: nine were prospective RCTs and four were kinetic studies (**Table 1**). The RCTs were analyzed in a metaanalysis,[59] in which the investigators concluded that EPO treatment decreased the need for RBC transfusions in critically ill patients (over all studies, odds ratio (OR): .73 [.64–.84, 95 % confidence interval (CI)], P<.001), except for a study by Corwin and colleagues.[54] The overall mean number of RBC units transfused per patient was decreased by .41 units per patient; EPO administration had no effect on 28-day mortality (over all studies, OR: .86 [.71–1.05, 95 % CI], P = .14).

Nevertheless, there are several flaws present in most of these studies. First, almost all of the studies relied on the synergistic effects of the association of iron and EPO on bone marrow production that has been reported in patients with terminal kidney failure. This principle was used in all studies realized in critically ill patients except for a pharmacokinetic study from Arroliga and colleagues,[56] in which iron administration was at the discretion of the investigators, and the retrospective study of Brophy and colleagues,[57] in which 48% of the patients received EPO combined with iron (see **Table 1**). No studies have compared the effects on hemoglobin levels of administration of EPO and iron to those of EPO alone in critically ill patients. But, because of the potential side effects of iron therapy (immunomodulation, ileus, abdominal pain, infections), studies on EPO administration without iron may be interesting. Nevertheless, the problem of sustaining iron stores during stimulated erythropoiesis by EPO remains, although this argument is relatively minor because of the few doses administered in critically ill patients (maximum five doses). Moreover, no studies reported iron kinetics during EPO therapy in critically ill patients, except the study by van Iperen and colleagues[41] comparing iron alone to EPO plus iron. In 12 patients, these

**Table 1**
Studies on EPO therapy in critically ill patients

| Name | Type of Study | Number and Type of Patients Treated With EPO | Transfusion Policy | Principal Results |
|---|---|---|---|---|
| Still et al, 1995[48] | MRCT | 19 patients with second- and third-degree burns of 25% to 65% total body surface | No policy. | No differences in Hb, Hct, reticulocyte count, serum iron, total iron binding capacity, transfusion requirements, or mortality. Increased DVT. |
| Gabriel et al, 1998[49] | SRCT | 9 surgical or trauma patients with MOF | To maintain Hct >30 %. | Increased reticulocyte count. |
| Corwin et al,1999[50] | MRCT | 80 anemic medicosurgical patients (Hct <38%) | No policy. | Increased Hct and decreased cumulative RBC transfusion. No difference in mortality or side effects. |
| van Iperen et al, 2000[41] | SRCT | 12 anemic medical ICU patients (Hb <11.2 g/dL or <12.1 g/dL in case of cardiac disease) | Transfusion standardized at an Hb concentration of 8.9 g/dL, in cases of a cardiac history at 9.7 g/dL, or when clinically necessary. | Increased serum EPO, reticulocyte count, serum transferrin receptors. |
| Corwin et al, 2002[51] | MRCT | 650 anemic medicosurgical patients (Hct <38 %) | No RBC transfusion if Hb ≥9 g/dL or Hct ≥27%, unless there was a specific clinical indication. RBC transfusion for Hb <9 g/dL or Hct <27% was at physician's discretion. | Increased Hb and decreased need for RBC transfusion and RBC transfusion per day alive. No effects on mortality or side events. |

| Georgopoulos et al, 2005[52] | MRCT | 100 medicosurgical anemic patients (Hb <12 g/dL) | Transfusion at Hb of 7 g/dl and, in cases of active cardiac ischemia and central nervous system damage, at 9 g/dl. No threshold of Hb if bleeding. | EPO increased the Hct in relation to the dose used. Decreased need for RBC transfusion, related to the dose of EPO. No difference in incidence of serious adverse events. |
| Silver et al, 2006[53] | MRCT | 42 patients in long-term acute care (Hct <38%) | No RBC transfusion for Hct ≥ 24%, unless there was a specific clinical indication (active bleeding, ischemia, or other) RBC transfusion for Hct <24 % at physician's discretion. | Decreased need for RBC transfusion at 42 days but not at 84 days. No difference in mortality and side effects. |
| Vincent et al, 2006[42] | MRCT | 44 medicosurgical anemic patients (Hct <38%) | No policy. | Increased EPO and reticulocyte count. No decreased RBC transfusion. |
| Corwin et al, 2007[54] | MRCT | 733 medicosurgical anemic patients (Hb <12 g/dL) | The need for RBC transfusion was determined by each patient's treating physician. RBC transfusion was targeted to maintain an Hb between 7–9 g/dL; unless there was a specific clinical indication (eg, active bleeding or ischemia). | No decreased RBC transfusion. No effect on mortality except patients with trauma. Increased DVT incidence. |

(continued on next page)

**Table 1**
*(continued)*

| Name | Type of Study | Number and Type of Patients Treated With EPO | Transfusion Policy | Principal Results |
|---|---|---|---|---|
| Talving et al, 2010[55] | Matched case control study | 89 brain trauma patients | No policy. | Decreased in-hospital mortality. |
| Arroliga et al, 2009[56] | Randomized, multicenter, open-label | 60 medicosurgical anemic patients separated into different regimens of EPO (Hb ≤12 g/dL) | No policy. | Increased peak of reticulocytes after 11 and 15 days. Same evolution independent of the EPO regimen. |
| Brophy GM et al, 2008[57] | Retrospective, multicenter, observational study | 438 medicosurgical anemic patients (Hb before the first dose of EPO: 9.2 [1.2] mean [SD]) | No policy. | Decreased need for RBC transfusion. Increase of Hb by 0.8 g/dL. 50% of patients did not receive ICU and hospital transfusions after the first dose of EPO. Length of therapy 1 week in 50% of patients. |
| Napolitano et al, 2010[58] | Post hoc analysis of two MRCTs[51,54] | 402 anemic trauma patients (Hct ≤38 %) | The need for RBC transfusion was determined by each patient's treating physician. RBC transfusion was targeted to maintain an Hb between 7–9 g/dL; unless there was a specific clinical indication (eg, active bleeding or ischemia). | Decreased mortality independent of the severity of the trauma. Increased thrombotic events. |

*Abbreviations:* DVT, deep vein thrombosis; Hb, hemoglobin concentration; Hct, hematocrit; MOF, multiple organ failure; MRCT, multicenter randomized controlled trial; SRCT, single center randomized controlled trial.

investigators observed significantly increased transferrin saturation with EPO associated with iron compared with iron alone, without changes in iron or ferritin concentrations. This result argues in favor of a stimulated bone marrow.

Second, the EPO used was always epoetin alfa (short half-life), and no RCTs were performed with an EPO with a longer half-life (eg, darbepoetin alfa). Pharmacokinetic data for the different EPOs are shown in **Table 2**. Because of the lower EPO concentrations after several days of ICU stay and perhaps reduced inflammatory syndrome,[45] it would perhaps be interesting to use glycosylated EPO to optimize bone marrow production.

Third, the dose used for epoetin alfa in these trials was very large, from 300 or 600 U/kg for 3 or 5 days to 40,000 units per week (see **Tables 1** and **2**), and the method of administration was different among studies or among patients in the same study (intravenous or subcutaneous). Additionally, no measurements of antierythropoietin antibodies were reported in the studies. Although these immunologic abnormalities remain rare, this information is important if we are to generalize the administration of EPO in critically ill patients.[60]

Fourth, EPO administration increased hematocrit values (the desired effect) but also increased blood viscosity (adverse effect). This adverse effect could favor the development of deep venous thrombosis. None of the studies reported a systematic search for this complication or for other thrombotic events during the study period. Only three of the studies in **Table 1** reported other cardiovascular events (hypertension, stroke, and so forth).

Fifth, as reported in other trials in critically ill patients, patients with heterogeneous pathologic conditions were included in these large trials (see **Table 1**). Only the study by Corwin and colleagues[54] reported subgroups analyses that were defined a priori, yet because of the pleiotropic effects of EPO, it is perhaps interesting to study patients with particular pathologic conditions (sepsis, trauma, brain injury, and so forth). In a subgroup of 402 trauma patients, Corwin and colleagues[54] reported decreased mortality in the EPO group at 29 days (OR, .37; 95% CI, .19–.72) and at 140 days (OR, .40; 95% CI, .23–.69). Analysis of trauma patients from the first and second EPO RCTs[51,54] showed the same beneficial effects on mortality after adjustment for the baseline characteristics and severity of trauma.[58] Nevertheless, these results were challenged by the increased adverse effects of EPO therapy in the second trial (clinically relevant thrombosis events: 16% vs 13%, relative risk: 1.3, 95% CI: .93–1.85).[54]

Sixth, EPO was started in these large trials if the hematocrit value was below 38% (see **Table 1**). The question is, was this not too early? Except for the early anemia described by Claessens and colleagues[47] and decreased iron utilization by the bone marrow and a marked inflammatory state, may it not be better to wait before starting EPO until, for example, the hematocrit value is less than 30%? Moreover, the primary end point of these studies was the decrease in RBC transfusions during the study period. Six of the nine randomized controlled trials reported a policy for RBC transfusion during the period of the study, but not all used a restrictive strategy (see **Table 1**). Because of the worldwide trend to limit RBC transfusions, this end point is perhaps no longer ideal. The negative trial for this end point by Corwin and colleagues[54] is perhaps a good example.

### Pleiotropic Effects of EPO

The decreased mortality at days 29 and 140 in trauma patients treated with EPO[51,54,58] may be explained by the pleiotropic effects of EPO, especially in the brain.[61] EPO increases RBC lifespan through the Janus tyrosine kinase 2 (Jak-2)

**Table 2**
Pharmacokinetic studies of EPO in critically ill patients

| Drug | Type of EPO | Posology | Route of Administration | Mean Terminal Half-Life (h) | References |
|---|---|---|---|---|---|
| Epoetin alfa | r-HuEPO | 40,000 U/wk maximum 4 doses | SC | At day 1 : 23.8 ± 11.9 At day 8 : 23.8 ± 13.7 | Vincent et al[42] |
| | | 40,000 U/wk maximum 3 doses | SC | | Corwin et al[51] |
| | | 40,000 U/wk maximum 3 doses | SC | | Corwin et al[54] |
| | | 300 U/kg day 3 to day 7, 150 U/kg per day from day 7 to day 30 | IV | | Still et al[48] |
| | | 300 U/kg on day 1,3,5,7,9 | SC | | van Iperen et al[41] |
| | | 40,000 U/wk maximum 2 doses | IV | 9.5 ± 2.4 | Arroliga et al[56] |
| | | 40,000 U/wk maximum 2 doses | SC | 24.5 ± 5.5 | |
| | | 40,000 U/wk + 15000 U each day until day 15 | IV | | |
| | | 40,000 U/wk + 15,000 U each day until day 15 | SC | | |
| | | 40,000 U/wk | SC | | Georgopoulos et al[52] |
| | | 40,000 U/three times a week, maximum 3 doses | SC | | |
| | | 300 U/kg day 3 to day 42 | SC | | Corwin et al[50] |
| | | 600 U/kg three times per week | IV | | Gabriel et al[49] |
| Darbepoetin alfa | Glycosylated EPO | 100 to 150 µg once weekly | IV and SC | | Brophy et al[57] |

*Abbreviations:* IV, intravenous; r-HuEPO, recombinant human EPO; SC, subcutaneous.

pathway after binding to a specific cell surface receptor (EpoR). This EpoR is widely expressed in the brain, retina, heart, kidney, smooth muscle cells, myoblasts, and vascular endothelium, suggesting pluripotent effects in normal health and pathologic conditions.[62] Several inflammatory cytokines increase expression of EpoR, including insulin-like growth factor, IL-1$\beta$, IL-6, and TNF-$\alpha$, suggesting a higher avidity of the EPO receptor during inflammation.[63] The probable beneficial effects reported with EPO may be due to antiapoptotic effects in neuronal, renal, endothelial, and cardiovascular systems. Indeed, several studies have reported decreased apoptosis and organ damage in animal models of ischemia/reperfusion.[64,65]

If EPO is produced locally in the brain in response to acute hypoxia and protects neurons against neuromediator-induced neurotoxicity,[66,67] exogenous recombinant EPO could cross the blood-brain barrier and ameliorate angiogenesis in an injured brain. Nevertheless, utilization of EPO for stroke in clinical trials was associated with conflicting results. The Göttingen EPO stroke study observed a better neurologic outcome and improved magnetic resonance imaging scan at 1 month in patients with stroke who received EPO therapy (100,000 U during 3 days), without deleterious effects.[68] However, a later study with combined administration of EPO and tissue-plasminogen activator reported no advantage.[69]

EPO may also have potentially beneficial effects after cardiac ischemia. Xenocostas and colleagues[70] reported the same reduction in infarct size with high dose EPO therapy (2000 U/kg) as with transfusion of fresh RBCs in anemic rats. These morphologic advantages were associated with decreased cardiomyocyte apoptosis and preserved left cardiac function in this group of rats. However, extrapolation of these data to humans has been disappointing. Three RCTs with EPO in patients with myocardial infarction showed no or very limited improvements in left ventricular function and no improvement in infarct size.[71–73]

Interestingly, EPO also has potentially beneficial effects on the microcirculation and may thereby improve cellular biochemistry during sepsis.[74,75] Kao and colleagues[74] observed that administration of EPO (400 U/kg) for 18 hours after sepsis induced by cecal ligature and perforation ameliorated the peritoneal microcirculation and muscular NADH (reduced, or hydrogenated, nicotinamide adenine dinucleotide) accumulation suggesting improvement in mitochondrial complex I function. These improvements, combined with the antiinflammatory (for example, decreased TNF and IL-1)[76] and cytoprotective (for example, increased protection against superoxide dismutase and thus synthesis of reactive oxygen species)[77] effects of EPO could make EPO an interesting therapy in sepsis.

## SUMMARY

Iron and EPO, alone or together, are two erythropoietic stimulating agents that could limit the development of anemia and reduce RBC transfusions in critically ill patients. More data on physiopathology, time course of alterations, and thresholds or markers to decide whether and when to use or stop these agents are lacking. Because of the risk of increasing bacterial growth and thus infection with iron administration, just one RCT was found in the literature. The results of this study were exciting, but studies assessing the time course of hepcidin during iron supplementation are needed before iron can be more widely used in critically ill patients. Because of their less marked inflammatory status and less severe depression of bone marrow iron utilization, nonseptic ICU patients probably remain the best candidates for iron supplementation.

Several trials have been conducted with EPO administration, but the RCTs performed so far have been too heterogeneous to provide convincing information. EPO compounds with longer half-lives may be more appropriate in ICU patients and, because of the restrictive RBC transfusion practice used worldwide in critically ill patients, the primary end point of decreased RBC transfusions is probably no longer appropriate. The pleiotropic effects of EPO and, especially, decreased apoptosis, may offer interesting uses for this hormone in critically ill patients. There are still too few data to support iron and EPO use in critically ill patients. Further large RCTs are needed.

## ACKNOWLEDGMENTS

The authors are sincerely grateful to C. Danguy, Pharm, from the Department of Pharmacy, CHU-Charleroi, for her help in preparing the tables for the manuscript.

## REFERENCES

1. WHO Scientific Group on Nutritional Anemias. Nutritional anemias: report of a WHO Scientific Group. Geneva (Switzerland): World Health Organization; 1968. Available at: http://whqlibdoc.who.int/trs/WHO_TRS_405.pdf. Accessed April 30, 2012.
2. Guralnik JM, Eisenstaedt RS, Ferrucci L, et al. Prevalence of anemia in persons 65 years and older in the United States: evidence for a high rate of unexplained anemia. Blood 2004;104:2263–8.
3. Vincent JL, Baron JF, Reinhart K, et al. Anemia and blood transfusion in critically ill patients. JAMA 2002;288:1499–507.
4. Corwin HL, Gettinger A, Pearl RG, et al. The CRIT Study: anemia and blood transfusion in the critically ill--current clinical practice in the United States. Crit Care Med 2004;32:39–52.
5. Walsh TS, Garrioch M, Maciver C, et al. Red cell requirements for intensive care units adhering to evidence-based transfusion guidelines. Transfusion 2004;44:1405–11.
6. Carson JL, Poses RM, Spence RK, et al. Severity of anaemia and operative mortality and morbidity. Lancet 1988;1:727–9.
7. Mudumbai SC, Cronkite R, Hu KU, et al. Association of admission hematocrit with 6-month and 1-year mortality in intensive care unit patients. Transfusion 2011;51: 2148–59.
8. Bateman AP, McArdle F, Walsh TS. Time course of anemia during six months follow up following intensive care discharge and factors associated with impaired recovery of erythropoiesis. Crit Care Med 2009;37:1906–12.
9. Nguyen BV, Bota DP, Melot C, et al. Time course of hemoglobin concentrations in nonbleeding intensive care unit patients. Crit Care Med 2003;31:406–10.
10. Vincent JL, Piagnerelli M. Transfusion in the intensive care unit. Crit Care Med 2006;34:S96–101.
11. Corwin HL, Parsonnet KC, Gettinger A. RBC transfusion in the ICU. Is there a reason? Chest 1995;108:767–71.
12. Hebert PC, Wells G, Tweeddale M, et al. Does transfusion practice affect mortality in critically ill patients? Transfusion Requirements in Critical Care (TRICC) Investigators and the Canadian Critical Care Trials Group. Am J Respir Crit Care Med 1997;155: 1618–23.
13. Hebert PC, Wells G, Blajchman MA, et al. A multicenter, randomized, controlled clinical trial of transfusion requirements in critical care. Transfusion Requirements in Critical Care Investigators, Canadian Critical Care Trials Group. N Engl J Med 1999;340:409–17.

14. Hebert PC, Fergusson DA, Stather D, et al. Revisiting transfusion practices in critically ill patients. Crit Care Med 2005;33:7–12.
15. Netzer G, Liu X, Harris AD, et al. Transfusion practice in the intensive care unit: a 10-year analysis. Transfusion 2010;50:2125–34.
16. Carson JL, Terrin ML, Noveck H, et al. Liberal or restrictive transfusion in high-risk patients after hip surgery. N Engl J Med 2011;365:2453–62.
17. Westbrook A, Pettila V, Nichol A, et al. Transfusion practice and guidelines in Australian and New Zealand intensive care units. Intensive Care Med 2010;36: 1138–46.
18. Scharte M, Fink MP. Red blood cell physiology in critical illness. Crit Care Med 2003;31:S651–7.
19. Kemna E, Pickkers P, Nemeth E, et al. Time-course analysis of hepcidin, serum iron, and plasma cytokine levels in humans injected with LPS. Blood 2005;106:1864–6.
20. Theurl I, Theurl M, Seifert M, et al. Autocrine formation of hepcidin induces iron retention in human monocytes. Blood 2008;111:2392–9.
21. Theurl I, Aigner E, Theurl M, et al. Regulation of iron homeostasis in anemia of chronic disease and iron deficiency anemia: diagnostic and therapeutic implications. Blood 2009;113:5277–86.
22. Piagnerelli M, Vincent JL. Role of iron in anaemic critically ill patients: it's time to investigate! Crit Care 2004;8:306–7.
23. Weiss G, Goodnough LT. Anemia of chronic disease. N Engl J Med 2005;352: 1011–23.
24. Munoz M, Romero A, Morales M, et al. Iron metabolism, inflammation and anemia in critically ill patients. A cross-sectional study. Nutr Hosp 2005;20:115–20.
25. Patteril MV, Davey-Quinn AP, Gedney JA, et al. Functional iron deficiency, infection and systemic inflammatory response syndrome in critical illness. Anaesth Intensive Care 2001;29:473–8.
26. Bobbio-Pallavicini F, Verde G, Spriano P, et al. Body iron status in critically ill patients: significance of serum ferritin. Intensive Care Med 1989;15:171–8.
27. Piagnerelli M, Rapotec A, Cotton F, et al. Iron administration in the critically ill. Semin Hematol 2006;43(Suppl):S23–7.
28. Mumby S, Margarson M, Quinlan GJ, et al. Is bleomycin-detectable iron present in the plasma of patients with septic shock? Intensive Care Med 1997;23:635–9.
29. Ozment CP, Turi JL. Iron overload following red blood cell transfusion and its impact on disease severity. Biochim Biophys Acta 2009;1790:694–701.
30. Hod EA, Zhang N, Sokol SA, et al. Transfusion of red blood cells after prolonged storage produces harmful effects that are mediated by iron and inflammation. Blood 2010;115:4284–92.
31. Piagnerelli M, Cotton F, Herpain A, et al. Time course of iron metabolism in critically ill patients. Acta Clinica Belgica 2012. [Epub ahead of print.]
32. Rodriguez RM, Corwin HL, Gettinger A, et al. Nutritional deficiencies and blunted erythropoietin response as causes of the anemia of critical illness. J Crit Care 2001;16:36–41.
33. Pieracci FM, Barie PS. Diagnosis and management of iron-related anemias in critical illness. Crit Care Med 2006;34:1898–905.
34. Fernandez R, Tubau I, Masip J, et al. Low reticulocyte hemoglobin content is associated with a higher blood transfusion rate in critically ill patients: a cohort study. Anesthesiology 2010;112:1211–5.
35. Lasocki S, Longrois D, Montravers P, et al. Hepcidin and anemia of the critically ill patient: bench to bedside. Anesthesiology 2011;114:688–94.

36. Lasocki S, Millot S, Andrieu V, et al. Phlebotomies or erythropoietin injections allow mobilization of iron stores in a mouse model mimicking intensive care anemia. Crit Care Med 2008;36:2388–94.
37. Javadi P, Buchman TG, Stromberg PE, et al. High-dose exogenous iron following cecal ligation and puncture increases mortality rate in mice and is associated with an increase in gut epithelial and splenic apoptosis. Crit Care Med 2004;32:1178–85.
38. Hod EA, Brittenham GM, Billote GB, et al. Transfusion of human volunteers with older, stored red blood cells produces extravascular hemolysis and circulating non-transferrin-bound iron. Blood 2011;118:6675–82.
39. Brasseur A, Cotton F, Zouaoui K, et al. Effects of red blood cell transfusion on iron metabolism and oxidative stress in critically ill patients [abstract]. Transfus Alt Transfus Med 2010;11(Suppl 2):P21.
40. Agarwal R. Nonhematological benefits of iron. Am J Nephrol 2007;27:565–71.
41. van Iperen CE, Gaillard CA, Kraaijenhagen RJ, et al. Response of erythropoiesis and iron metabolism to recombinant human erythropoietin in intensive care unit patients. Crit Care Med 2000;28:2773–8.
42. Vincent JL, Spapen HD, Creteur J, et al. Pharmacokinetics and pharmacodynamics of once-weekly subcutaneous epoetin alfa in critically ill patients: results of a randomized, double-blind, placebo-controlled trial. Crit Care Med 2006;34:1661–7.
43. Pieracci FM, Henderson P, Rodney JR, et al. Randomized, double-blind, placebo-controlled trial of effects of enteral iron supplementation on anemia and risk of infection during surgical critical illness. Surg Infect (Larchmt) 2009;10:9–19.
44. Rogiers P, Zhang H, Leeman M, et al. Erythropoietin response is blunted in critically ill patients. Intensive Care Med 1997;23:159–62.
45. Elliot JM, Virankabutra T, Jones S, et al. Erythropoietin mimics the acute phase response in critical illness. Crit Care 2003;7:R35–R40.
46. Vialet R, Ventre C, Leone M, et al. Erythropoietin measurements in severely traumatized patients. Acta Anaesthesiol Scand 2008;52:601–4.
47. Claessens YE, Fontenay M, Pene F, et al. Erythropoiesis abnormalities contribute to early-onset anemia in patients with septic shock. Am J Respir Crit Care Med 2006;174:51–7.
48. Still JM Jr, Belcher K, Law EJ, et al. A double-blinded prospective evaluation of recombinant human erythropoietin in acutely burned patients. J Trauma 1995;38: 233–6.
49. Gabriel A, Kozek S, Chiari A, et al. High-dose recombinant human erythropoietin stimulates reticulocyte production in patients with multiple organ dysfunction syndrome. J Trauma 1998;44:361–7.
50. Corwin HL, Gettinger A, Rodriguez RM, et al. Efficacy of recombinant human erythropoietin in the critically ill patient: a randomized, double-blind, placebo-controlled trial. Crit Care Med 1999;27:2346–50.
51. Corwin HL, Gettinger A, Pearl RG, et al. Efficacy of recombinant human erythropoietin in critically ill patients: a randomized controlled trial. JAMA 2002;288:2827–35.
52. Georgopoulos D, Matamis D, Routsi C, et al. Recombinant human erythropoietin therapy in critically ill patients: a dose-response study [ISRCTN48523317]. Crit Care 2005;9:R508–R515.
53. Silver M, Corwin MJ, Bazan A, et al. Efficacy of recombinant human erythropoietin in critically ill patients admitted to a long-term acute care facility: a randomized, double-blind, placebo-controlled trial. Crit Care Med 2006;34:2310–6.
54. Corwin HL, Gettinger A, Fabian TC, et al. Efficacy and safety of epoetin alfa in critically ill patients. N Engl J Med 2007;357:965–76.

55. Talving P, Lustenberger T, Kobayashi L, et al. Erythropoiesis stimulating agent administration improves survival after severe traumatic brain injury: a matched case control study. Ann Surg 2010;251:1–4.

56. Arroliga AC, Guntupalli KK, Beaver JS, et al. Pharmacokinetics and pharmacodynamics of six epoetin alfa dosing regimens in anemic critically ill patients without acute blood loss. Crit Care Med 2009;37:1299–307.

57. Brophy GM, Sheehan V, Shapiro MJ, et al. A US multicenter, retrospective, observational study of erythropoiesis-stimulating agent utilization in anemic, critically ill patients admitted to the intensive care unit. Clin Ther 2008;30:2324–34.

58. Napolitano LM, Fabian TC, Kelly KM, et al. Improved survival of critically ill trauma patients treated with recombinant human erythropoietin. J Trauma 2008;65:285–97.

59. Zarychanski R, Turgeon AF, McIntyre L, et al. Erythropoietin-receptor agonists in critically ill patients: a meta-analysis of randomized controlled trials. CMAJ 2007;177: 725–34.

60. Casadevall N, Nataf J, Viron B, et al. Pure red-cell aplasia and antierythropoietin antibodies in patients treated with recombinant erythropoietin. N Engl J Med 2002; 346:469–75.

61. Patel NS, Collino M, Yaqoob MM, et al. Erythropoietin in the intensive care unit: beyond treatment of anemia. Ann Intensive Care 2011;1:40.

62. Arcasoy MO. The non-haematopoietic biological effects of erythropoietin. Br J Haematol 2008;141:14–31.

63. Walden AP, Young JD, Sharples E. Bench to bedside: a role for erythropoietin in sepsis. Crit Care 2010;14:227.

64. Malese K, Li F, Chong ZZ. New avenues of exploration for erythropoietin. JAMA 2005;293:90–5.

65. Sepodes B, Maio R, Pinto R, et al. Recombinant human erythropoietin protects the liver from hepatic ischemia-reperfusion injury in the rat. Transpl Int 2006;19:919–26.

66. Siren AL, Knerlich F, Poser W, et al. Erythropoietin and erythropoietin receptor in human ischemic/hypoxic brain. Acta Neuropathol 2001;101:271–6.

67. Brines ML, Ghezzi P, Keenan S, et al. Erythropoietin crosses the blood-brain barrier to protect against experimental brain injury. Proc Natl Acad Sci U S A 2000;97: 10526–31.

68. Ehrenreich H, Hasselblatt M, Dembowski C, et al. Erythropoietin therapy for acute stroke is both safe and beneficial. Mol Med 2002;8:495–505.

69. Ehrenreich H, Weissenborn K, Prange H, et al. Recombinant human erythropoietin in the treatment of acute ischemic stroke. Stroke 2009;40:e647–56.

70. Xenocostas A, Hu H, Chin-Yee N, et al. Erythropoietin is equally effective as fresh-blood transfusion at reducing infarct size in anemic rats. Crit Care Med 2010;38: 2215–21.

71. Voors AA, Belonje AM, Zijlstra F, et al. A single dose of erythropoietin in ST-elevation myocardial infarction. Eur Heart J 2010;31:2593–600.

72. Najjar SS, Rao SV, Melloni C, et al. Intravenous erythropoietin in patients with ST-segment elevation myocardial infarction: REVEAL: a randomized controlled trial. JAMA 2011;305:1863–72.

73. Ott I, Schulz S, Mehilli J, et al. Erythropoietin in patients with acute ST-segment elevation myocardial infarction undergoing primary percutaneous coronary intervention: a randomized, double-blind trial. Circ Cardiovasc Interv 2010;3:408–13.

74. Kao R, Xenocostas A, Rui T, et al. Erythropoietin improves skeletal muscle microcirculation and tissue bioenergetics in a mouse sepsis model. Crit Care 2007;11:R58.

75. Kao RL, Martin CM, Xenocostas A, et al. Erythropoietin improves skeletal muscle microcirculation through the activation of eNOS in a mouse sepsis model. J Trauma 2011;71:S462–S467.
76. Cuzzocrea S, Di PR, Mazzon E, et al. Erythropoietin reduces the development of nonseptic shock induced by zymosan in mice. Crit Care Med 2006;34:1168–77.
77. Mitra A, Bansal S, Wang W, et al. Erythropoietin ameliorates renal dysfunction during endotoxaemia. Nephrol Dial Transplant 2007;22:2349–53.

# Transfusion Reactions
## Newer Concepts on the Pathophysiology, Incidence, Treatment, and Prevention of Transfusion-Related Acute Lung Injury

David M. Sayah, MD, PhD[a],*, Mark R. Looney, MD[b], Pearl Toy, MD[c]

KEYWORDS

- Transfusion-related acute lung injury • Acute lung injury • Transfusion reaction
- Multiple transfusions • Pulmonary edema

KEY POINTS

- Transfusion-related acute lung injury (TRALI), a form of acute lung injury (ALI) that develops shortly after blood product transfusion, is the leading cause of transfusion-related mortality.
- The development of TRALI is influenced by both transfusion-related and patient-related risk factors, which have now been identified.
- Diagnosis of TRALI requires a high index of suspicion and is based on the exclusion of cardiogenic pulmonary edema, sepsis from a bacteria-contaminated blood product, and other causes of acute lung injury.
- Treatment of TRALI is largely supportive and is similar to that of other forms of ALI.
- TRALI incidence can be reduced by reducing the transfusion of plasma from previously pregnant donors.

## INTRODUCTION

Since 2003, the leading cause of transfusion-related fatality has been transfusion-related acute lung injury (TRALI),[1] defined as acute lung injury (ALI)[2] that develops

Grant support: The project described was supported by National Heart, Lung, and Blood Institute Transfusion Medicine SCCOR P50HL081027 (P.T.), HL107386 (M.R.L.) and HL007185 (D.M.S.).
[a] Division of Pulmonary, Critical Care, Allergy and Sleep Medicine, Department of Medicine, University of California, San Francisco, Box 0130, San Francisco, CA 94143–0130, USA; [b] Division of Pulmonary, Critical Care, Allergy and Sleep Medicine, Department of Medicine and Laboratory Medicine, University of California, San Francisco, San Francisco, CA, USA; [c] Department of Laboratory Medicine, University of California, San Francisco, Box 0451, San Francisco, CA 94143–0451, USA
* Corresponding author.
E-mail address: David.Sayah@ucsf.edu

Crit Care Clin 28 (2012) 363–372
http://dx.doi.org/10.1016/j.ccc.2012.04.001
0749-0704/12/$ – see front matter © 2012 Elsevier Inc. All rights reserved.

---

**Box 1**
**Summary of National Heart, Lung, and Blood Institute consensus working group definition of TRALI**

**Development of ALI, defined as**

- Acute onset.

- Hypoxemia ($Pao_2/Fio_2$ Ratio $\leq$300 mm Hg).

- Bilateral pulmonary opacities on frontal chest radiograph.

- Absence of left atrial hypertension (pulmonary artery occlusion pressure $\leq$18 mm Hg if measured).

**In patients <u>without</u> other ALI risk factors:**

- New onset of ALI during or within 6 hours after the end of transfusion of a plasma-containing blood product.

**In patients <u>with</u> other ALI risk factors:**

- New onset of ALI during or within 6 hours after the end of transfusion of a plasma-containing blood product.

- Clinical course suggestive of TRALI—the ALI is not attributable to the ALI risk factor, and the patient was clinically stable before transfusion.

*Adapted from* Toy P, Popovsky MA, Abraham E, et al. Transfusion-related acute lung injury: Definition and review. Crit Care Med 2005;33(4):721–6; and Bernard GR, Artigas A, Brigham KL, et al. The American-European Consensus Conference on ARDS. Definitions, mechanisms, relevant outcomes, and clinical trial coordination. Am J Respir Crit Care Med 1994;149(3 Pt 1):818–24.

---

during or within 6 hours after transfusion of 1 or more units of blood or blood components.[3,4] Included in this definition are cases of ALI after multiple transfusions, a well-known ALI risk factor.[5] The condition has been underreported since the first description by Popovsky and colleagues.[6] In the United States, the incidence of TRALI before 2007 is estimated at 1 in 4000 to 1 in 5000 units transfused,[7,8] although preventative measures (described later) may have reduced this incidence to 1 in 12,000 by 2009.[8] TRALI mortality has been estimated at approximately 6%,[7] considerably lower than the estimated mortality of other forms of ALI/acute respiratory distress syndrome (ARDS).[9]

## DEFINITION OF TRALI

TRALI is defined as new ALI that develops during or within 6 hours of transfusion of 1 or more units, not attributable to another ALI risk factor (**Box 1**).[4] To diagnose patients with the highest likelihood of TRALI, patients who concurrently have another major ALI risk factor (pneumonia, sepsis, aspiration, multiple fractures, and pancreatitis) are usually excluded. Such patients are labeled possible TRALI[3] or transfused ALI.[8]

## PATHOPHYSIOLOGY

The pathogenesis of TRALI has usually been explained by the transfusion of a blood product that contains anti–human leukocyte antigen (anti-HLA) or anti–human neutrophil antigen (anti-HNA) antibodies that recognize cognate antigen in the transfusion recipient. Case series have documented the presence of such antibodies and their cognate antigens in TRALI patients,[7] and animal models of TRALI have been developed that use anti-major histocompatibility class I or anti-HNA antibodies to promote TRALI.[10,11] In these experimental models of TRALI, allorecognition by such antibodies leads to neutrophil-dependent ALI, characterized by robust neutrophilic inflammation of the lung and disruption of the lung alveolar-capillary permeability barrier, similar to what is seen in other forms of ALI/ARDS.[10,11] A role for monocytes has also been implicated.[12,13] Furthermore, activated platelets have also been shown to play a pathogenic role in experimental models of TRALI, likely via interactions with neutrophils.[14,15]

Despite the substantial evidence implicating transfused antibodies in the pathogenesis of TRALI, uncertainty remains. One important observation is that cognate antibodies are not detected in all clinically diagnosed cases of TRALI.[7,8] Experimental models have implicated biologically active lipids in the pathogenesis of TRALI that develops in the absence of antileukocyte antibodies.[16,17] Such lipids have been shown to be breakdown products of cell membrane phospholipids that form during prolonged storage of cellular blood components.[18] In particular, lysophosphatidylcholine, has been identified as a component of such blood products that can prime neutrophils. However, a case-control study in cardiac surgery patients[19] and a recent large case-control study in general transfused patients failed to demonstrate an association between such biologically active lipids (as well as other bioreactive substances including soluble CD40 ligand), and an increased risk of TRALI.[8] In addition, nonpolar lipids in the plasma of stored leukoreduced red blood cells also prime neutrophils in vitro, but the clinical relevance of this observation remains to be determined.[20]

A second important observation is that not all recipients transfused with a blood product containing a matched anti-HLA or anti-HNA antibody develop evidence of TRALI. Thus, it is likely that factors other than transfusion of any of these antibodies are capable of initiating TRALI, and that cofactors, related either to the transfused product or to the recipient, are important in the pathogenesis of antibody-mediated TRALI. These observations have led to a multiple-event hypothesis of TRALI pathogenesis, which states that a transfusion recipient must have an underlying medical condition or conditions that, likely via immune priming, lead to a susceptibility to TRALI that is then triggered by the transfusion of alloantibody or other bioreactive substances.[21] This multievent hypothesis is supported by animal models in which antibody-induced TRALI develops only when there is a preexisting inflammatory stimulus, and by case-control human studies of TRALI risk factors (described later).[8,14]

## TRALI RISK FACTORS
### Risk of Greater Number of Transfusions

TRALI has long been known to be associated with multiple transfusions.[5] In a case-control study, increased number of transfusions was associated with increased risk, which was partially explained by transfusion and patient risk factors identified by multivariate analysis.[8]

### Transfusion Risk Factors

Although all blood components have been implicated in TRALI, three strong predictors of TRALI risk by multivariate analysis are receipt of female plasma or whole blood, larger quantity of strong cognate anti-HLA-Class II (HLA class II antibody) (cognate is defined as antibody specificity that matches recipient antigen), and larger volume of anti-HNA.[8] Multiparous females can be alloimmunized and produce antileukocyte antibodies,[22] explaining the higher risk of TRALI associated with blood products from female donors.

Regarding the relative importance of Class I versus Class II HLA antibody, Class II is more important.[8] The association of HLA Class II antibodies with TRALI was first reported by Kopko and colleagues.[23] Case series have reported cognate anti-HLA-Class II was the most frequent antibody implicated in TRALI.[24,25] This predominance occurs despite the fact that frequencies of Class I (10%) and Class II (12%) antibodies are comparable in female donors.[22]

Regarding class I HLA antibody, there is evidence against anti-HLA-Class I (HLA class I antibody) being an important risk, even for strong cognate antibody with mean fluorescent intensity (MFI) greater than 2500.[8] Others have reported similar results[26] and similar conclusions.[27] There are reports that cognate anti-HLA-Class I can be associated with TRALI.[24,25,28] However, studies of previous recipients of blood from donors implicated in TRALI have found that this is rare.[29,30]

Often in previous studies and current practice, the finding of any cognate HLA antibody or HNA (human neutrophil antigens) antibody in any transfused unit has been considered presumptive evidence of TRALI, regardless of antibody strength or volume. A case-control study suggests, however, that with a multivariate analysis of risk factors, cognate anti-HLA-Class I and weak cognate anti-HLA-Class II have little or no impact on TRALI risk.[8]

Bioreactive substances in blood units did not seem to be associated with substantial risk in two clinical studies.[8,19] This result was surprising, given many basic studies that indicate bioreactive substances are important in the development of TRALI.[17,31,32]

Why do some patients develop TRALI and others who receive blood from the same donor do not? Cognate antibody matters,[8] and patients who developed TRALI may have received cognate antibody and others did not. However, cognate versus noncognate antibody is not the only reason, because several studies of previous recipients of blood from implicated donors have found patients who received cognate antibody but did not develop TRALI.[29,30,33] Three additional factors influence why some patients develop TRALI and others do not: first, the quantity of cognate antibody transfused (antibody strength times volume of plasma containing the antibody), second, the class of the HLA antibody, and third, the presence or absence of patient factors that increase the risk for TRALI.[8]

### Patient Risk Factors

By multivariate analysis in a case-control study, patient risk factors are[8]

- Higher interleukin-8 (IL-8) level
- Shock
- Liver surgery (mainly transplantation)
- Chronic alcohol abuse
- Positive fluid balance
- Peak airway pressure greater than 30 cm $H_2O$ if mechanically ventilated before transfusion
- Current smoking.

The diverse patient-associated risk factors are consistent with the known underlying comorbidities that predispose and lower the threshold for ALI, thus supporting the validity of these results. Shock results in tissue injury,[34] perhaps predisposing to TRALI through priming of the recipient's endothelium and immune cells. Chronic alcohol abuse increases risk, likely due to reduced levels of the antioxidant glutathione in the lung,[35] reduced phagocytosis of apoptotic cells, and the resulting enhanced pulmonary inflammatory response.[36] Patients with intravascular volume

---

**Box 2**
**ALI risk factors**

- Septic shock

- Sepsis syndrome without hypotension

- Aspiration of gastric contents

- Near-drowning

- Disseminated intravascular coagulation

- Pulmonary contusion

- Pneumonia requiring ICU care

- Drug overdose requiring ICU care

- Fracture of long bones or pelvis

- Burn, any percent of body surface

- Cardiopulmonary bypass

*Abbreviation:* ICU, intensive care unit.

*Adapted from* Toy P, Popovsky MA, Abraham E, et al. Transfusion-related acute lung injury: definition and review. Crit Care Med 2005;33(4):721–26.

---

overload are more likely to manifest clinical pulmonary edema when there is ALI.[37] Previous studies have documented the risk for developing ALI with peak airway pressure greater than 30 cm $H_2O$[38] and current smoking.[39,40]

Higher levels of IL-8, a marker of inflammation and increased mortality risk,[41] may prime neutrophils and the lung endothelium. Acute contemporaneous events that increase inflammation and tissue injury could be "first hits" as first suggested by Silliman and colleagues.[17] Experimental models of TRALI have shown that host inflammation may be necessary to produce ALI before challenge with cognate antibody.[14,31] Inflammation (first hit) may upregulate expression of HLA Class II antigens on classic antigen presenting cells (macrophages, dendritic cells), activated neutrophils,[42] and activated lung endothelial cells,[43] and exposure to large quantities of strong HLA Class II cognate antibody may then lead to ALI (second hit).[44] Whereas first hit traditionally refers to neutrophil priming usually associated with inflammation in the recipient,[17] it is now known that additional recipient conditions predispose patients to TRALI.[8] These are general factors that predispose a patient to any form of ALI. Thus, it is reasonable to revise and broaden the concept of first hit in the multiple-event model of TRALI to include not only conditions that result in neutrophil priming, but also patient conditions that predispose to and reduce the threshold for ALI.

## CLINICAL MANIFESTATIONS AND DIAGNOSIS

TRALI is underrecognized, and making the diagnosis requires a high index of suspicion. The diagnosis of TRALI is based on clinical findings of ALI manifested within 6 hours of receiving a blood product transfusion, in the absence of another risk factor for the development of lung injury (see **Box 1**; **Box 2**). TRALI commonly develops well prior to the 6-hour time point, often during the first hour of a transfusion. Clinical hallmarks of TRALI include:

- Dyspnea
- Tachypnea
- Hypoxemia
- Bilateral pulmonary opacities on chest radiograph
- Edema fluid in the endotracheal tube of intubated patients (severe TRALI)
- Absence of evidence of volume overload or cardiac dysfunction as the principal cause of pulmonary edema.

Febrile reactions as well as hypothermia have been reported in patients with TRALI, as have both hypotension and hypertension.

In mechanically ventilated patients, the diagnosis should be considered whenever there is an acute, unexplained worsening in respiratory status that is temporally associated with a transfusion. In such patients, copious frothy pink edema fluid is often recovered from the endotracheal tube. The differential diagnosis includes cardiogenic pulmonary edema, including transfusion-associated circulatory overload, and other causes of ALI/ARDS. In the context of a recent transfusion and the absence of other apparent risk factors for ALI/ARDS, the exclusion of cardiogenic pulmonary edema strongly supports the diagnosis of TRALI.

Whereas there are no specific diagnostic tests for TRALI, several common clinical tests can be used to support the diagnosis:

- Echocardiogram
- Brain natriuretic peptide (BNP)
- Pulmonary edema fluid protein analysis
- White blood cell (WBC) count.

Echocardiography, measurement of the BNP level, and analysis of pulmonary edema fluid are useful and complementary tests in helping to exclude cardiac dysfunction and volume overload. Echocardiography can be particularly helpful by providing insight into both cardiac function and volume status. BNP can similarly be used to help exclude volume overload. If undiluted pulmonary edema fluid is collected along with a matched plasma sample, the presence of a permeability pulmonary edema can be established, which generally excludes cardiogenic edema.[45] Whereas pulmonary artery catheterization and determination of pulmonary artery occlusion pressure provide additional information regarding volume status, routine use of this invasive procedure is not warranted. Transient leukopenia has been temporally associated with the onset of TRALI, and serial measurements of WBC may reveal this finding.[46] Whereas none of these adjunctive tests are specific for TRALI, in the right clinical context they can build a clinical case for the diagnosis.

In addition to the supportive clinical diagnostic tests previously described, confirmatory laboratory testing can provide definitive evidence for the diagnosis of TRALI by investigating for the presence of transfused cognate antibodies. The blood bank should be notified of all cases of suspected TRALI so that other components from the same involved donation can be quarantined. Donor retention specimens in the blood bank or donor recall samples should be used for antibody testing. A patient blood sample should be saved for HLA antigen testing, should strong HLA Class II antibody be found in an involved donor. However, as discussed previously, it is important to note that cognate antileukocyte antibodies are not found in all cases of TRALI and that the diagnosis of TRALI is ultimately based on the clinical scenario and the exclusion of other diagnoses.

In a TRALI patient with fever and hypotension, it is important to rapidly exclude the possibility of ALI associated with sepsis due to the transfusion of bacteria-contaminated platelets. The diagnosis is made by a positive gram stain of the residual contents of the transfused platelet unit and by identification of the same organism in blood cultures of the patient and culture of the involved platelet unit.

## TREATMENT

As with other forms of ALI/ARDS, there is no specific treatment for TRALI. In most cases, TRALI is self-limited and carries a better prognosis than other causes of ALI/ARDS. However, prompt diagnosis allows for the implementation of proper supportive care, which is generally the same as for any patient with ALI/ARDS. In addition, potentially harmful interventions, such as the administration of diuretics, should be avoided. In fact, patients with TRALI who are hypotensive may require intravenous fluids to maintain an adequate blood pressure.

If the patient is still being transfused when the diagnosis is first suspected, the transfusion should be stopped immediately. For mild cases, supplemental oxygen and routine supportive care may be sufficient. For severe cases, mechanical ventilation, intravenous fluids, invasive hemodynamic monitoring, and vasopressors may be required. In rare cases the hypoxemia resulting from TRALI can be so severe that extracorporeal oxygenation may be required as a temporizing measure while the lungs heal.[47,48] In patients who require mechanical ventilation, a low tidal volume strategy, as would be used in other cases of ALI/ARDS, should be used.[38] Whereas several case reports describe the treatment of TRALI with glucocorticoids, no randomized, controlled trials have studied this therapy in TRALI. Given the potential complications associated with glucocorticoids, and the typically self-limited course of TRALI, there is no clear role for glucocorticoids in the treatment of TRALI.

## PREVENTION

Receipt of female plasma (including whole blood) is a strong risk factor, and reduction of this risk factor in 2007 to 2008 was concurrent with a decrease in TRALI incidence determined by active surveillance at two academic medical centers from year 2006 to 2009 from approximately 1 in 4,000 units to approximately 1 in 12,000 units.[8] The premitigation incidence of approximately 1 in 4,000 units found in 2006 was close to the approximately 1 in 5,000 units found by a careful study at the Mayo Clinic where a transfusion team performed and monitored transfusions,[7] but 10-fold higher than the 2005 premitigation incidence of approximately 1 in 40,000 units distributed found by passive surveillance (26.3 cases in $10^6$ units).[49] Decreases in TRALI after conversion to male-predominant plasma have been reported by passive surveillance studies from the United Kingdom,[50] the US Food and Drug Administration,[1] and the American Red Cross.[51] Patient factors likely contributed to the decrease in incidence, for example, institutional improvements in critical care delivery that reduce patient risk factors that seem to render patients susceptible to TRALI,[19] such as improving treatment of septic shock and decreasing high peak airway pressure greater than 30 cm $H_2O$ while being mechanically ventilated.

The American Association of Blood Banks recommended the reduction of the transfusion of plasma and platelets from probable high-risk donors.[52,53] The decrease in TRALI observed after implementation of such programs supports the effectiveness of this approach. To further reduce TRALI risk in female plasma-rich components, clinical evidence supports the suggested screening for strong anti-HLA-Class II in platelet donors[54] and the development of high-throughput granulocyte immunofluorescence test methods to screen for known and unknown human neutrophil antigens.[8] In addition, reduction of modifiable patient risk factors should also reduce the risk for developing TRALI.

## REFERENCES

1. Fatalities reported to FDA following blood collection and transfusion: annual summary for fiscal year 2009. Annual Summaries 2010. Available at: http://www.fda.gov/BiologicsBloodVaccines/SafetyAvailability/ReportaProblem/TransfusionDonationFatalities/ucm204763.htm. Accessed February 2, 2011.
2. Bernard GR, Artigas A, Brigham KL, et al. The American-European Consensus Conference on ARDS. Definitions, mechanisms, relevant outcomes, and clinical trial coordination. Am J Respir Crit Care Med 1994;149(3 Pt 1):818–24.
3. Kleinman S, Caulfield T, Chan P, et al. Toward an understanding of transfusion-related acute lung injury: statement of a consensus panel. Transfusion 2004; 44(12):1774–89.
4. Toy P, Popovsky MA, Abraham E, et al. Transfusion-related acute lung injury: Definition and review. Crit Care Med 2005;33(4):721–6.
5. Fowler AA, Hamman RF, Good JT, et al. Adult respiratory distress syndrome: risk with common predispositions. Ann Intern Med 1983;98(5 Pt 1):593–7.
6. Popovsky MA, Abel MD, Moore SB. Transfusion-related acute lung injury associated with passive transfer of antileukocyte antibodies. Am Rev Respir Dis 1983;128(1): 185–9.
7. Popovsky MA, Moore SB. Diagnostic and pathogenetic considerations in transfusion-related acute lung injury. Transfusion 1985;25(6):573–7.
8. Toy P, Gajic O, Bacchetti P, et al. Transfusion related acute lung injury: incidence and risk factors. Blood 2012;119(7):1757–67.
9. Rubenfeld GD, Caldwell E, Peabody E, et al. Incidence and outcomes of acute lung injury. N Engl J Med 2005;353(16):1685–93.
10. Looney MR, Su X, Van Ziffle JA, et al. Neutrophils and their Fc gamma receptors are essential in a mouse model of transfusion-related acute lung injury. J Clin Invest 2006;116(6):1615–23.
11. Sachs UJ, Hattar K, Weissmann N, et al. Antibody-induced neutrophil activation as a trigger for transfusion-related acute lung injury in an ex vivo rat lung model. Blood 2006;107(3):1217–9.
12. Sachs UJ, Wasel W, Bayat B, et al. Mechanism of transfusion-related acute lung injury induced by HLA class II antibodies. Blood 2011;117(2):669–77.
13. Strait RT, Hicks W, Barasa N, et al. MHC class I-specific antibody binding to nonhematopoietic cells drives complement activation to induce transfusion-related acute lung injury in mice. J Exp Med 2011;208(12):2525–44.
14. Looney MR, Nguyen JX, Hu Y, et al. Platelet depletion and aspirin treatment protect mice in a two-event model of transfusion-related acute lung injury. J Clin Invest 2009;119(11):3450–61.
15. Hidalgo A, Chang J, Jang JE, et al. Heterotypic interactions enabled by polarized neutrophil microdomains mediate thromboinflammatory injury. Nat Med 2009;15(4): 384–91.
16. Silliman CC, Voelkel NF, Allard JD, et al. Plasma and lipids from stored packed red blood cells cause acute lung injury in an animal model. J Clin Invest 1998;101(7): 1458–67.
17. Silliman CC, Bjornsen AJ, Wyman TH, et al. Plasma and lipids from stored platelets cause acute lung injury in an animal model. Transfusion 2003;43(5):633–40.
18. Silliman CC, Clay KL, Thurman GW, et al. Partial characterization of lipids that develop during the routine storage of blood and prime the neutrophil NADPH oxidase. J Lab Clin Med 1994;124(5):684–94.

19. Vlaar AP, Hofstra JJ, Determann RM, et al. The incidence, risk factors, and outcome of transfusion-related acute lung injury in a cohort of cardiac surgery patients: a prospective nested case-control study. Blood 2011;117(16):4218–25.

20. Silliman CC, Moore EE, Kelher MR, et al. Identification of lipids that accumulate during the routine storage of prestorage leukoreduced red blood cells and cause acute lung injury. Transfusion 2011;51(12):2549–54.

21. Silliman CC, Paterson AJ, Dickey WO, et al. The association of biologically active lipids with the development of transfusion-related acute lung injury: a retrospective study. Transfusion 1997;37(7):719–26.

22. Triulzi DJ, Kleinman S, Kakaiya RM, et al. The effect of previous pregnancy and transfusion on HLA alloimmunization in blood donors: implications for a transfusion-related acute lung injury risk reduction strategy. Transfusion 2009;49(9):1825–35.

23. Kopko PM, Popovsky MA, MacKenzie MR, et al. HLA class II antibodies in transfusion-related acute lung injury. Transfusion 2001;41(10):1244–8.

24. Reil A, Keller-Stanislawski B, Gunay S, et al. Specificities of leucocyte alloantibodies in transfusion-related acute lung injury and results of leucocyte antibody screening of blood donors. Vox Sang 2008;95(4):313–7.

25. Chapman CE, Stainsby D, Jones H, et al. Ten years of hemovigilance reports of transfusion-related acute lung injury in the United Kingdom and the impact of preferential use of male donor plasma. Transfusion 2009;49(3):440–52.

26. Gajic O, Rana R, Winters JL, et al. Transfusion-related acute lung injury in the critically ill: prospective nested case-control study. Am J Respir Crit Care Med 2007;176(9): 886–91.

27. Bierling P, Bux J, Curtis B, et al. Recommendations of the ISBT Working Party on Granulocyte Immunobiology for leucocyte antibody screening in the investigation and prevention of antibody-mediated transfusion-related acute lung injury. Vox Sang 2009;96(3):266–9.

28. Dykes A, Smallwood D, Kotsimbos T, et al. Transfusion-related acute lung injury (Trali) in a patient with a single lung transplant. Br J Haematol 2000;109(3):674–6.

29. Cooling L. Transfusion-related acute lung injury. JAMA 2002;288(3):315–6.

30. Toy P, Hollis-Perry KM, Jun J, et al. Recipients of blood from a donor with multiple HLA antibodies: a lookback study of transfusion-related acute lung injury. Transfusion 2004;44(12):1683–8.

31. Kelher MR, Masuno T, Moore EE, et al. Plasma from stored packed red blood cells and MHC class I antibodies causes acute lung injury in a 2-event in vivo rat model. Blood 2009;113(9):2079–87.

32. Silliman CC, Boshkov LK, Mehdizadehkashi Z, et al. Transfusion-related acute lung injury: epidemiology and a prospective analysis of etiologic factors. Blood 2003; 101(2):454–62.

33. Muniz M, Sheldon S, Schuller RM, et al. Patient-specific transfusion-related acute lung injury. Vox Sang 2008;94(1):70–3.

34. Blennerhassett JB. Shock lung and diffuse alveolar damage pathological and pathogenetic considerations. Pathology 1985;17(2):239–47.

35. Moss M, Guidot DM, Wong-Lambertina M, et al. The effects of chronic alcohol abuse on pulmonary glutathione homeostasis. Am J Respir Crit Care Med 2000;161 (2 Pt 1):414–9.

36. Boe DM, Richens TR, Horstmann SA, et al. Acute and chronic alcohol exposure impair the phagocytosis of apoptotic cells and enhance the pulmonary inflammatory response. Alcohol Clin Exp Res 2010;34:1723–32.

37. Wiedemann HP, Wheeler AP, Bernard GR, et al. Comparison of two fluid-management strategies in acute lung injury. N Engl J Med 2006;354(24):2564–75.

38. Ventilation with lower tidal volumes as compared with traditional tidal volumes for acute lung injury and the acute respiratory distress syndrome. The Acute Respiratory Distress Syndrome Network. N Engl J Med 2000;342(18):1301–8.
39. Iribarren C, Jacobs DR Jr, Sidney S, et al. Cigarette smoking, alcohol consumption, and risk of ARDS: a 15-year cohort study in a managed care setting. Chest 2000; 117(1):163–8.
40. Calfee CS, Matthay MA, Eisner MD, et al. Active and passive cigarette smoking and acute lung injury after severe blunt trauma. Am J Respir Crit Care Med 2011;183(12): 1660–5.
41. Parsons PE, Eisner MD, Thompson BT, et al. Lower tidal volume ventilation and plasma cytokine markers of inflammation in patients with acute lung injury. Crit Care Med 2005;33(1):1–6 [discussion: 230–2].
42. Gosselin EJ, Wardwell K, Rigby WF, et al. Induction of MHC class II on human polymorphonuclear neutrophils by granulocyte/macrophage colony-stimulating factor, IFN-gamma, and IL-3. J Immunol 1993;151(3):1482–90.
43. Geppert TD, Lipsky PE. Antigen presentation by interferon-gamma-treated endothelial cells and fibroblasts: differential ability to function as antigen-presenting cells despite comparable Ia expression. J Immunol 1985;135(6):3750–62.
44. Kopko PM, Paglieroni TG, Popovsky MA, et al. TRALI: correlation of antigen-antibody and monocyte activation in donor-recipient pairs. Transfusion 2003;43(2):177–84.
45. Yost CS, Matthay MA, Gropper MA. Etiology of acute pulmonary edema during liver transplantation: a series of cases with analysis of the edema fluid. Chest 2001;119(1): 219–23.
46. Looney MR, Gropper MA, Matthay MA. Transfusion-related acute lung injury: a review. Chest 2004;126(1):249–58.
47. Lee AJ, Koyyalamudi PL, Martinez-Ruiz R. Severe transfusion-related acute lung injury managed with extracorporeal membrane oxygenation (ECMO) in an obstetric patient. J Clin Anesth 2008;20(7):549–52.
48. Kuroda H, Masuda Y, Imaizumi H, et al. Successful extracorporeal membranous oxygenation for a patient with life-threatening transfusion-related acute lung injury. J Anesth 2009;23(3):424–6.
49. Eder A, Herron R, Strupp A, et al. Transfusion-related acute lung injury surveillance (2003–2005) and the potential impact of the selective use of plasma from male donors in the American Red Cross. Transfusion 2007;47(4):599–607.
50. SHOT Annual Reports and Summaries (All). SHOT 2010. Available at: http://www.shotuk.org/wp-content/uploads/2011/07/SHOT-2010-Report1.pdf. Accessed August 6, 2011.
51. Eder AF, Herron RM Jr, Strupp A, et al. Effective reduction of transfusion-related acute lung injury risk with male-predominant plasma strategy in the American Red Cross (2006–2008). Transfusion 2010;50(8):1732–42.
52. Transfusion-related acute lung injury. AABB Association Bulletin 2006. Available at: http://www.aabb.org/Content/Members_Area/Association_Bulletins/ab06-07.htm. Accessed February 2, 2011.
53. Clarifications to recommendations to reduce the risk of TRALI. AABB Association Bulletin 2007. Available at: htp://http://www.aabb.org/Content/Members_Area/Association_Bulletins/ab07-03.htm. Accessed February 2, 2011.
54. Carrick DM, Norris PJ, Endres RO, et al. Establishing assay cutoffs for HLA antibody screening of apheresis donors. Transfusion 2011;51(10):2092–101.

# The Utility of a Diagnostic Scoring System for Disseminated Intravascular Coagulation

Satoshi Gando, MD, PhD, FCCM

## KEYWORDS

- Disseminated intravascular coagulation • Diagnosis • Score • Critical illness

## KEY POINTS

- DIC should be recognized as a serious condition that should be diagnosed and treated as early as possible in the critical care setting.
- Three diagnostic scoring systems for DIC published by the ISTH, the JAAM, and the JMHW are now available.
- It would be better to select the scoring system based on a full understanding of the diagnostic properties.

From the early 1970s to 1980s, several disseminated intravascular coagulation (DIC) diagnostic criteria were published.[1–3] At that time, there was already recognition of the clinical importance of DIC, and DIC was also called "Death Is Coming."[2] However, no universally accepted definition or diagnostic algorithm for DIC has existed until recently. In 1988, the Japanese Ministry of Health and Welfare (JMHW) proposed a scoring system for DIC by revising their 1983 version of the criteria.[3,4] The Scientific Standardization Committee (SSC) of the International Society on Thrombosis and Haemostasis (ISTH) subsequently announced overt and nonovert DIC scoring systems partly based on the 1988 JMHW scoring system in the early 2000s.[5] In this communication, the ISTH also provided a clear and universally accepted definition of DIC for the first time. During the 1990s, structural and functional studies clarified the tight interplay between coagulation and inflammation.[6,7] These studies supported an important role of systemic inflammatory response syndrome (SIRS) in the development of DIC in critically ill patients.[7,8] DIC in turn contributes to the development of

No conflict of interest to disclose.

Division of Acute and Critical Care Medicine, Department of Anesthesiology and Critical Care Medicine, Hokkaido University Graduate School of Medicine, N15W7, Kita-ku, Sapporo 060–8638, Japan

E-mail address: gando@med.hokudai.ac.jp

Crit Care Clin 28 (2012) 373–388

http://dx.doi.org/10.1016/j.ccc.2012.04.004

multiple organ dysfunction syndrome (MODS) and its complications in this patient group associated with SIRS.[9] Based on this evidence and referring to the previous criteria, the Japanese Association for Acute Medicine (JAAM) DIC study group developed a new DIC scoring system for critically ill patients.[10,11] Both the ISTH and the JAAM DIC scoring systems have been prospectively validated, and their usefulness in various clinical situations, including the critical care setting, has been confirmed.[10-13] Although some comments on these have been proposed,[14] clinical comparisons for these criteria have been published.[15] Recently, two guidelines and one expert consensus about the DIC diagnosis and its treatment of DIC have been announced from three societies of thrombosis and hemostasis.[16-18] Comments for these guidelines have also been proposed.[19-21]

Based on this historical background, this review discusses the need for better methods for diagnosing DIC, laboratory tests used for the diagnosis of DIC, and finally, the diagnostic scoring system for DIC that can be used in the critical care setting.

## THE NEED FOR A BETTER METHOD FOR DIAGNOSING OF DIC
### The Need for a Treatment for DIC

Although most clinicians are aware of the general conditions resulting from DIC, a precise description of the syndrome and a good working definition and useful scoring system were not available until recently. Therefore, in spite of the fact that DIC was sometimes referred to as "Death Is Coming" by hematologists, most critical care physicians considered that DIC was merely the endpoint of organ dysfunction and it was ignored as an epiphenomenon associated with various serious illnesses in the early 1990s. For this reason, DIC was not considered a disease or syndrome to be treated. Consequently, precise diagnostic tools were not considered to be necessary for the management of DIC.

**Fig. 1**A shows the different causes and results of primary and secondary MODS proposed by the American College of Chest Physicians and the Society of Critical Care Medicine (ACCP/SCCM) in the early 1990s.[6] Primary organ dysfunction is the direct result of an insult in which organ dysfunction occurs early and is directly attributable to the insult itself. Secondary MODS develops as a consequence of excessive host responses and is identified in the context of SIRS. Therefore, to prevent secondary MODS, in addition to the insult itself, simultaneous treatments for excessive host response are needed. At the time of the ACCP/SCCM proposal, however, most physicians believed that only inflammatory cytokine-induced SIRS reflected the host responses to infectious (eg, sepsis) and noninfectious (eg, trauma) insults. Based on this concept, anticytokine strategies to control systemic inflammation were considered to benefit patients with SIRS.[22] However, all of the antiinflammatory strategies designed to treat insults such as sepsis during the 1990s failed.[23] In the mid-1990s, a new concept, the interaction between coagulation and inflammation, was developed. Physicians then started to think that in addition to the insult, the excessive inflammation and pathologic activation of coagulation (DIC) should be treated simultaneously.[7-9,24]

The presence of DIC increases the chance of mortality beyond that associated with the primary insult.[25] Additionally, the removal of the insult that caused DIC does not necessarily alleviate the DIC process; restoration of coagulation abnormalities and organ dysfunction take some time.[16,26] Dhainaut and colleagues[27] demonstrated that coagulopathy preceded the MODS and that continued coagulopathy during the first day of severe sepsis increases the risk of new organ dysfunction and death. Through the subgroup analyses of large-scale randomized control trials, it was demonstrated

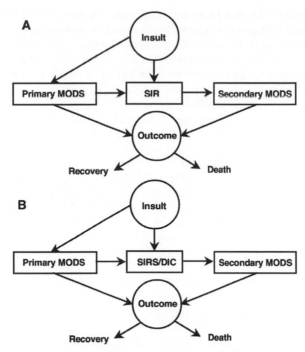

**Fig. 1.** The knowledge about the different causes and results of primary and secondary MODS. (*A*) During the early 1990s, the systemic inflammatory response (SIR) mediating the excessive host response was thought to cause secondary MODS. (*B*) After recognition of the close interplay between inflammation and coagulation, recently it is believed that SIRS and DIC originated from systemic inflammation synergistically causing secondary MODS. (*From* Members of the American College of Chest Physicians/Society of Critical Care Medicine Consensus Conference committee. American College of Chest Physicians/Society of Critical Care Medicine Consensus Conference: definitions for sepsis and organ failure and guidelines for the use innovative therapies in sepsis. Crit Care Med 1992;20:864–74; with permission.)

that treatment of DIC with drugs possessing both antiinflammatory and anticoagulation properties improved the prognosis of severe sepsis and septic shock associated with DIC.[28,29] These studies supported the need for simultaneous treatment of inflammation and DIC in addition to the inciting insult (eg, sepsis) itself. Therefore, DIC was recognized as a syndrome that needs to be treated, and the new treatment paradigm is depicted in **Fig. 1**B.

### The Need for a Standard Definition and Diagnosis of DIC

In order for treatments to be developed for DIC, there was a need for a precise definition of the condition and widely accepted diagnostic criteria. It had long been recognized that DIC is not a disease in itself, but is a syndrome that always develops secondary to an underlying disorder. DIC is characterized by the inflammatory cytokine-initiated activation of tissue factor–dependent coagulation, insufficient control of coagulation by physiologic anticoagulation pathways, and plasminogen activator inhibitor-1 (PAI-1)-mediated attenuation of fibrinolysis.[9] Collectively, these changes result in the widespread formation of fibrin thrombosis, microvascular occlusion, and reduced oxygen delivery to cells and tissues, leading to MODS.[30]

During the process of activation of coagulation, subsequent consumption and exhaustion of platelets and coagulation factors lead to bleeding and hemorrhage into tissues, so-called consumption coagulopathy.[5,9] Considering these characteristics of DIC, the SSC of the ISTH proposed a definition for DIC as, "DIC is an acquired syndrome characterized by the intravascular activation of coagulation with loss of localization arising from different causes. It can originate from and cause damage to the microvasculature, which if sufficiently severe, can produce organ dysfunction."[5]

In the previous subgroup studies, the ISTH overt and nonovert DIC scoring systems can select proper patient groups who need DIC treatments.[28,29] The JMHW diagnostic criteria for DIC were also used for randomized controlled trials of a new anticoagulant, recombinant soluble thrombomodulin for DIC, and its utility was demonstrated.[31] More important, Wada and colleagues[32] confirmed that starting the treatment of DIC at the early stage when the JMHW DIC scores were still low had a greater impact on improving the patient prognosis and that the outcome became poorer when the treatment was begun when the DIC scores were higher. These results suggest that early diagnosis and early treatment based on the DIC scoring system are important for improving the patient outcome. These studies illustrated the utility of the diagnostic scoring system for DIC in various clinical settings, including critical care. DIC can thus be recognized to be an independent syndrome, and it should be differentially diagnosed from similar coagulopathies by its definition and diagnostic criteria.

## LABORATORY TESTS FOR THE DIC DIAGNOSTIC SCORING SYSTEM

There has been no single test that is sufficiently accurate to establish or rule out a diagnosis of DIC. Therefore, the diagnostic scoring system for DIC uses a combination of several laboratory tests.[33,34] Because DIC is a dynamic process that varies with time, the disease parameters should always be repeatedly evaluated based on the sequential monitoring of readily available and inexpensive laboratory tests that can be measured in laboratories worldwide.

### Assessment of the Platelet Count and Global Markers for Coagulation and Fibrinolysis

Platelets are sensitive to thrombin, and its generation can activate platelets, leading to a reduction of platelet counts due to adhesion-based and aggregation-based consumption. Low platelet counts and a reduction in the platelet counts over several measurements are a sensitive sign of DIC.[5,35] The development of thrombocytopenia comes late in the course of experimental models of sepsis[35]; however, in the clinical setting, platelet counts decline at an early phase of sepsis, and the platelet count is a very sensitive marker of DIC, especially in patients with sepsis. It is necessary to be aware that because of the wide distribution of normal counts, the platelet counts may remain within the normal range during the early stage of DIC. In this situation, a continuous drop or the rate of decrease for the platelet counts in consecutive measurements is more important for diagnosing DIC than are the absolute values.[10] Another important point is that thrombocytopenia is a relatively common hematologic problem seen in a wide variety of critically ill patients.[36] At the diagnosis of DIC, other causes of thrombocytopenia due to bone marrow suppression, an increased degree of destruction due to immune causes, dilution, and distribution to organs such as the spleen, should be carefully ruled out.[10,36]

Because of the methods used to measure them, the prothrombin time (PT) and activated partial thromboplastin time (APTT) do not accurately reflect in vivo hemostasis.[34] However, low levels of coagulation factors occurring due to their consumption are reflected by prolongation of the PT and APTT. The APTT represents the function of the intrinsic coagulation pathway including Factor VIII (FVIII), which is known to paradoxically increase in most DIC patients, probably due to the release of von Willebrand factor from the endothelium and the acute phase behavior of FVIII [33,34] Therefore, the APTT is sometimes normal or even shortened in spite of prolongation of the PT in patients with DIC. In critically ill patients, impaired synthesis of coagulation factors due to liver dysfunction or vitamin K deficiency and the presence of an inhibitory antibody can modify the values of PT and APTT. Although the specificity of PT and APTT for a DIC diagnosis is therefore relatively low, most DIC scoring systems adopt simple, rapid, and inexpensive PT and APTT tests.[3–5,10] The international normalized ratio (INR) has been used for the standardization of PT by evaluating the intensity of vitamin K antagonist.[37] However, because the INR was validated only for this purpose, it is not appropriate to apply the INR as a screening test for coagulation abnormalities such as DIC. However, the SSC on DIC of the ISTH recently published an official comment about the application of the INR in the scoring system for DIC.[38] In this report, the SSC concluded that use of plasma from patients with DIC to calibrate the PT-INR could result in improved comparability, and presumably reproducibility, of results using different commercial thromboplastins.

A low level of fibrinogen reflects a late, severe consumptive stage of DIC, because fibrinogen is an acute phase reactant and will remain falsely normal or even higher than normal during the early stage of DIC. Yu and colleagues[39] showed a low sensitivity (22%) and high specificity (100%) of fibrinogen in the diagnosis of DIC. Sequential monitoring of fibrinogen or revision of fibrinogen values by inflammatory markers such as C-reactive protein might therefore be more useful for the diagnosis of DIC.

Different from the previously mentioned markers of consumption, tests for fibrin degradation products such as fibrin/fibrinogen degradation products (FDP) and D-dimer, show direct evidence of thrombin-mediated fibrin thrombosis and its degradation by plasmin. Increased levels of FDP and D-dimer thus both indicate that the coagulation and fibrinolytic systems are activated, and that thrombin and plasmin have been generated. However, the available assays for FDP cannot discriminate between degradation products of cross-linked fibrin and fibrinogen. In contrast, D-dimer differentiates the degradation of cross-linked fibrin from fibrinogen and fibrinogen degradation products. Considering the nature of FDP and D-dimer, elevation of these markers in DIC is always necessary to confirm the diagnosis of DIC. In addition, extremely high levels of FDP and D-dimer can be observed in DIC associated with hyperfibrinolysis (DIC with fibrinolytic subtype), such as acute promyelocytic leukemia (APL).[40] In DIC associated with APL, the degree of FDP and D-dimer elevation is often disproportionate to the prolongation of PT and APTT and to the severity of thrombocytopenia. An enhanced expression of annexin II on the APL cells has been reported to induce hyperfibrinolysis.[40] In contrast, in DIC with higher PAI-1 levels (DIC with thrombotic phenotype), especially those associated with sepsis, a minor to moderate increase in the FDP and D-dimer levels is commonly observed due to the attenuation in fibrinolysis caused by elevated levels of PAI-1. In this type of DIC, the activation of the fibrinolytic system is insufficient to counteract the systemic activation of coagulation, which is thought to be one of the main causes of MODS in DIC.[9,34,41,42] The use of both FDP and D-dimer offered the best test panel with high sensitivity and moderate specificity for the diagnosis of DIC.[39] However, diseases such as deep vein thrombosis, recent trauma, and surgery associated with high levels of FDP and D-dimer should always be carefully ruled out. Moreover, poor standardization and harmonization, and different cutoffs that are not interchangeable among the different commercial assays available on the market, make the choice of the most predictive threshold for D-dimer expression difficult.[33]

### Molecular Markers

Thrombin-induced fibrin formation and the subsequent plasmin-mediated fibrin degradation play pivotal roles in the pathogenesis of DIC. After this role was recognized, numerous molecular markers were developed for detection of thrombin generation (prothrombin fragment 1+2), thrombin generation and its neutralization (thrombin antithrombin complex, TAT), thrombin activation (soluble fibrin, fibrinopeptide A), and for the detection of plasmin generation and its neutralization (plasmin antiplasmin complex) and for plasmin activation (fibrinopeptide B$\beta$15-42). Bick[43] presented an algorithm for the diagnosis of DIC using these molecular markers. Several studies proposed the possibility of using molecular markers for the diagnosis of DIC under various conditions; however, their specificity was low in spite of their high sensitivity.[44–46] In the clinical setting, these sensitive markers are generally already elevated during the course of SIRS without DIC, and they continue to rise as inflammation progresses, reaching their highest levels when DIC becomes prominent. For this reason, the ISTH suggested that molecular markers constitute important means for diagnosing nonovert DIC and that serial measurement of these parameters are important to assess the progression from nonovert to overt DIC.[5] In practice, however, these tests are beyond the scope of the routine diagnostic laboratory, are cost-consuming, and are therefore unrealistic for rapid and repeated measurements in the critical care setting. At this time, the practical use of molecular markers in clinical medicine is very limited.[34] The ISTH overt DIC and the JAAM DIC diagnostic scoring systems have not adopted the molecular markers for their scoring systems.

### THE DIAGNOSTIC SCORING SYSTEM FOR DIC

Scoring systems for DIC, developed from the JMHW scoring system, have been independently proposed by the ISTH and the JAAM.[3–5,10] The most striking difference in the latter two systems from the JMHW scoring system is a deletion of the points for underlying disorders, bleeding symptoms, and thrombosis-related organ dysfunction. Instead of adding one point for underlying disorders, the ISTH criterion added a table of "clinical conditions that may be associated with DIC" as a mandatory clause, and restricted the use of the scoring algorithm without the underlying diseases. The JAAM presents the same table, while also adding another table of "clinical conditions that should be carefully ruled out" in order to increase the specificity of the scoring system. The ISTH and the JAAM decided not to include the clinical assessment of bleeding symptoms and organ dysfunction as a part of the score, because the DIC score itself forms part of the scores associated with these two conditions.[5,10] The ISTH scoring system consists of overt and nonovert DIC criteria to identify the harbingers of DIC that progress to uncompensated and full-blown DIC. The ISTH suggested that treatments are most effective when nonovert DIC is present.[5,47,48]

The JAAM excluded the concept of nonovert or pre-DIC, and thereby intentionally increased the sensitivity of the scoring system to ensure the early diagnosis and immediate treatment of DIC as soon as a diagnosis has been made.[10,11] To put it concretely, the JAAM examined total-score diagnosing of DIC for two total points scores (4 and 5). A total score of 4 points could diagnose DIC earlier and more sensitively than a score of 5 points without changing the diagnostic properties or resulting in a different mortality for the patients. In accordance with these results, the JAAM adopted a total score of 4 points for a diagnosis of DIC.[10] Inclusion of the SIRS criteria, and the addition of a decreased platelet count rate to the scoring system and the removal of fibrinogen from the scoring system, are other features associated with the JAAM DIC scoring system. The study from the

ISTH also demonstrated that exclusion of all fibrinogen levels from the calculation of the ISTH scoring system hardly affected the accuracy of the scoring system.[12] Scoring systems are successful if clinicians can use them at the bedside, if they are readily available, and if they are easy to use. The criteria should be simple so that clinicians will be able to remember the criteria and easily apply them in the clinical setting. Therefore, all three criteria, the JMHW, the ISTH, and the JAAM, consist of assays of global markers of coagulation and fibrinolysis that are commonly available at all hospitals.

Whereas the absence of a 100% accurate gold standard for the diagnosis of DIC is a serious limitation, the three scoring systems have been prospectively and retrospectively compared in various clinical settings.[10,11,15,49–51] The results of these studies can be summarized as follows: (1) all of the scoring systems are useful for the diagnosis of DIC and predict a poor patient outcome; (2) the ISTH scoring system has a high specificity, whereas the JAAM scoring system has high sensitivity for the recognition of DIC; (3) the JAAM scoring system is useful for selecting DIC patients for early treatment; and (4) the JAAM DIC progresses to the ISTH overt DIC. At this point, it seems that the JAAM DIC score identifies a high-risk group of patients, some of whom also fulfill the more restrictive criteria of the ISTH and the JMHW DIC scores. It is conceivable that clinical deterioration will result in an increase in the proportion of patients fulfilling the ISTH and the JMHW criteria in the course of critical care treatments.[14,50] Finally, it should also kept in mind that all three criteria failed to discriminate between survivors and nonsurvivors among DIC patients associated with relatively low Acute Physiology and Chronic Health Evaluation (APACHE) II scores.[52–54] The relationships of the three DIC diagnostic scoring systems are presented in **Fig. 2**.

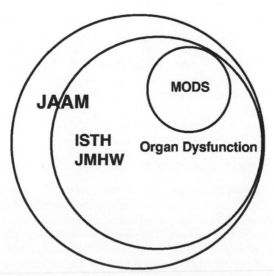

**Fig. 2.** The relationship between the ISTH, the JMHW, and the JAAM scoring systems for DIC. The ISTH and the JMHW scoring systems diagnose full-blown DIC that may be decompensated and associated with organ dysfunction or MODS. The JAAM DIC scoring system accurately diagnoses decompensated as well as compensated DIC, thus making it possible to achieve a different prognosis from the usual coagulopathy.

## THE ISTH OVERT AND NONOVERT DIC DIAGNOSTIC SCORING SYSTEM
### Overt DIC

**Table 1** shows the ISTH overt DIC scoring system.[5] The diagnostic accuracy of the ISTH score was evaluated in 217 consecutive patients suspected to have DIC who were admitted to the intensive care unit (ICU).[12] The study showed an acceptable accuracy for the diagnosis of DIC in critically ill patients with sepsis, severe sepsis, surgery, trauma, and so forth. The severity of DIC according to this scoring system is related to the mortality of patients with sepsis and other critical conditions.[28,29,55-57] Similar results were obtained from a retrospective study of children with sepsis.[58] However, the accuracy of the score for the other conditions associated with DIC, such as malignancy and obstetric disorders, has not yet been validated.[59,60]

The ISTH did not show clear cutoff values of the fibrin-related markers.[5] Instead, the ISTH recommends the use of three levels; no increase (0 point), a moderate increase (2 point) and a strong increase (3 point), depending on the type of test used. Dempfle and colleagues[61] recommended the use of soluble fibrin instead of D-dimer as the fibrin-related marker using cutoff values of the 25% and 75% quartiles of 1870 plasma samples from ICU patients for 2-point and 3-point scores. The subgroup analyses of large-scale randomized controlled trials[28,29] and a prospective validation study[12] used D-dimer as the fibrin-related marker, where a value above the upper limit of normal (.4–4.0 $\mu$g/mL) was considered a moderate increase, and a value higher than 10 times the upper limit of normal (>4.0 $\mu$g/mL) was considered a strong increase. Recent guidelines suggest that D-dimer should be the marker of choice, and recommended the use of these cutoff values.[18]

### Nonovert DIC

Using kinetic components and sensitive molecular markers, such as soluble fibrin and TAT, the ISTH proposed a scoring system for "nonovert DIC" that may detect the presence of hemostatic dysfunction when it is not yet at the stage of frank decompensation, namely overt DIC.[5] In contrast to this hypothesis, the prospective validation of a nonovert DIC scoring system demonstrated that the mortality of patients fulfilling the overt DIC and nonovert DIC criteria were similar, and progression of nonovert DIC to overt DIC was not observed.[61,62] These results suggest that nonovert DIC is independent of overt DIC, and that both the nonovert and overt criteria may miss the severe hemostatic changes associated with death. A combination of overt and nonovert scoring systems[14,29] or modifications of the nonovert scoring system[63,64] may improve the diagnostic capabilities of the nonovert DIC scoring system for compensated hemostatic changes.

## THE JAAM DIC DIAGNOSTIC SCORING SYSTEM

**Table 2** shows the JAAM DIC diagnostic scoring system.[10,11] The JAAM developed and published the JAAM DIC scoring system especially for critically ill patients based on problems discovered with the old JMHW scoring system, such as the low sensitivity for diagnosis and the lack of objective tools for scoring points associated with bleeding symptoms and thrombosis-related organ dysfunction.[10] Two prospective studies validated its clinical significance for the early and definite diagnosis of DIC in patients with critical illnesses.[10,11] A subgroup analysis of these two studies restricted for sepsis confirmed that the JAAM DIC patients exist in a dependent continuum with the ISTH overt DIC in septic patients, therefore enabling them to receive early treatment.[50] Sawamura and colleagues[65,66] demonstrated that the JAAM DIC diagnostic scoring system has acceptable validity for the diagnosis of DIC

**Table 1**
**The scoring system for overt DIC proposed by the ISTH**

Clinical conditions that may be associated with overt DIC:

- Sepsis/severe infection (any microorganism)
- Trauma (eg, polytrauma, neurotrauma, fat embolism)
- Organ dysfunction (eg, severe pancreatitis)
- Malignancy
  - Solid tumors
  - Myeloproliferative/lymphoproliferative malignancies
- Obstetric calamites
  - Amniotic fluid embolism
  - Abruptio placentae
- Vascular abnormalities
  - Kasabach-Merritt syndrome
  - Large vascular aneurysms
- Severe hepatic failure
- Severe toxic or immunologic reactions
  - Snakebite
  - Recreational drugs
  - Transfusion reactions
  - Transplant rejection

1. Risk assessment: Does the patient have an underlying disorder known to be associated with overt DIC?

   If yes: proceed; if no: do not use this algorithm.

2. Order global coagulation tests (platelet count, prothrombin time, soluble fibrin monomers, or fibrin degradation products).

3. Score global coagulation test results.

| • Platelet counts ($10^9$/L) | Score |
|---|---|
| <50 | 2 |
| ≥50 <100 | 1 |
| ≥100 | 0 |

| • Elevated fibrin-related marker (eg, soluble fibrin monomers/fibrin degradation products) | |
|---|---|
| Strong increase | 3 |
| Moderate increase | 2 |
| No increase | 0 |

| • Prolonged prothrombin time (s) | |
|---|---|
| ≥6 | 2 |
| ≥3 <6 | 1 |
| <3 | 0 |

| • Fibrinogen level (g/mL) | |
|---|---|
| <100 | 1 |
| ≥100 | 0 |

4. Calculate score

5. If >5: compatible with overt DIC; repeat scoring daily.

   If <5: suggestive (not affirmative) for nonovert DIC; repeat next 1–2 days.

**Table 2**
**The scoring system for DIC by the JAAM**

1. Clinical conditions that may be associated with DIC:

(1) Sepsis/severe infection (any microorganism)

(2) Trauma/burn/surgery

(3) Vascular abnormalities
  - Large vascular aneurysms
  - Giant hemangioma
  - Vasculitis

(4) Severe toxic or immunologic reactions
  - Snakebite
  - Recreational drugs
  - Transfusion reactions
  - Transplant rejection

(5) Malignancy (except bone marrow suppression)

(6) Obstetric calamities

(7) Conditions that may be associated with SIRS
  - Organ destruction (eg, severe pancreatitis)
  - Severe hepatic failure
  - Ischemia/hypoxia/shock
  - Heat stroke/malignant syndrome
  - Fat embolism
  - Rhabdomyolysis
  - Other

(8) Other

2. Clinical conditions that should be carefully ruled out:

A. Thrombocytopenia

(1) Dilution and abnormal distribution

Massive blood loss and transfusion, massive infusion

(2) Increased platelet destruction

ITP, TTP/HUS, HIT, drugs, viral infection, alloimmune destruction, APS, HELLP, extracorporeal circulation

(3) Decreased platelet production

Viral infection, drugs, radiation, nutritional deficiency (vitamin $B_{12}$, folic acid), disorders of hematopoiesis, liver disease, HPS

(continued on next page)

**Table 2**
*(continued)*

| | |
|---|---|
| (4) Spurious decrease | |
| EDTA-dependent agglutinins, insufficient anticoagulation of blood samples | |
| (5) Other | |
| Hypothermia, artificial devices in the vessel | |
| B. Prolonged prothrombin time | |
| Anticoagulation therapy, anticoagulant in blood samples, vitamin K deficiency, liver cirrhosis, massive blood loss and transfusion | |
| C. Elevated FDP | |
| Thrombosis, hemostasis and wound healing, hematoma, pleural effusion, ascites, anticoagulant in blood samples, antifibrinolytic therapy | |
| D. Other | |
| 3. The diagnostic algorithm for SIRS | |
| (1) Temperature >38°C or <36°C | |
| (2) Heart rate >90 beats/min | |
| (3) Respiratory rate >20 breaths/min or $PaCO_2$ <32 torr (<4.3 kPa) | |
| (4) White blood cell >12,000 cells/mm³, <4000 cells/mm³, or 10% immature (band) forms | |

4. The diagnostic algorithm

| | Score |
|---|---|
| SIRS criteria | |
| ≥3 | 1 |
| 0–2 | 0 |
| Platelet counts ($10^9$/L) | |
| <80 or more than 50% decrease within 24 h | 3 |
| ≥80 <120 or more than 30% decrease within 24 h | 1 |
| ≥120 | 0 |
| Prothrombin time (value of patient/normal value) | |
| ≥1.2 | 1 |
| <1.2 | 0 |
| Fibrin/fibrinogen degradation products (mg/L) | |
| ≥25 | 3 |
| ≥10 <25 | 1 |
| <10 | 0 |
| Diagnosis | |
| 4 points or more | DIC |

*Abbreviations:* APS, antiphospholipid syndrome; EDTA, ethylenediaminetetraacetic acid; HELLP, hemolysis, elevated liver enzymes, and low platelet; HIT, heparin-induced thrombocytopenia; HPS, hemophagocytic syndrome; HUS, hemolytic uremic syndrome; ITP, idiopathic thrombocytopenic purpura; $PaCO_2$, partial pressure of carbon dioxide, arterial; TTP, thrombotic thrombocytopenic purpura.

at an early phase of trauma, and that the scoring system can diagnose DIC with a higher sensitivity earlier than the ISTH overt DIC scoring system. Using DIC diagnosed with the obstetric DIC scoring system as the gold standard, the JAAM DIC scoring system was applied for the diagnosis of obstetric disorders.[67,68] The JAAM DIC scoring system could diagnose obstetric DIC with high sensitivity (94.7%) and moderate specificity (75.0%). The area under the receiver operating characteristic curve was .847 (95% confidence interval .740–.9555, $P = .0001$), which suggests that the JAAM DIC scoring system has an acceptable ability to diagnose obstetric DIC. Similar to the ISTH overt DIC scoring system, the accuracy of the JAAM DIC scoring system for the other conditions associated with DIC, such as malignancy, has not yet been validated.

## THE JMHW DIC DIAGNOSTIC SCORING SYSTEM

The JMHW DIC scoring system was first published two decades ago and has been widely used in both research and clinical investigations. However, its diagnostic accuracy has not been assessed until recently.[69] The JMHW DIC scoring system showed moderate sensitivity and high specificity for the diagnosis of DIC patients with hematologic malignancies; however, its usefulness for critically ill patients has not been validated. The diagnostic algorithm of the JMHW scoring system can be found elsewhere.[3,18,33] Future studies will be needed to assess its usefulness for patients with DIC associated with other conditions.

## SUMMARY

DIC is an acquired syndrome characterized by microvascular thrombosis as a result of the activation of coagulation, and it can produce organ dysfunction, leading to a poor prognosis for critically ill patients. Therefore, DIC should be recognized as a serious condition that should be diagnosed and treated as early as possible in the critical care setting. Prospectively validated DIC scoring systems with various diagnostic properties are now available for the DIC diagnosis. The selection of the particular DIC scoring system is dependent on the purpose of its application. For example, for the early diagnosis, the system with the higher sensitivity is needed, whereas a high specificity will be useful for confirming diagnosis.

Sustained SIRS is a warning sign of DIC, and a continuous decline in the platelet counts should be recognized as a condition that should be closely followed. After assessing the underlying disorders known to be associated with DIC, it is necessary to carefully rule out conditions that result in similar changes in laboratory data as are observed in cases of DIC. Daily repeated scoring is mandatory for both a definite diagnosis and to rule out DIC, as well as to characterize the severity and course of the DIC.

## REFERENCES

1. Colman RW, Robby SJ, Minna JD. Disseminated intravascular coagulation (DIC): an approach. Am J Med 1972;52:679–89.
2. Spero JA, Lewis JH, Hasiba U. Disseminated intravascular coagulation. Findings in 346 patients. Thromb Haemost 1980;43:28–33.
3. Kobayashi N, Maekawa T, Takada M, et al. Criteria for diagnosis of DIC based on the analysis of clinical and laboratory findings in 345 DIC patients collected by the Research Committee on DIC in Japan. Bibl Haematol 1983;49:265–75.
4. Wada H, Gabazza EC, Asakura H, et al. Comparison of diagnostic criteria for disseminated intravascular coagulation (DIC): diagnostic criteria of the International Society of Thrombosis and Haemostasis (ISTH) and of the Japanese Ministry of Health and Welfare for overt DIC. Am J Hematol 2003;74:17–22.

5. Taylor FB, Toh CH, Hoots WK, et al. Toward definition, clinical and laboratory criteria, and a scoring system for disseminated intravascular coagulation. Thromb Haemost 2001;86:1327–30.

6. Members of the American College of Chest Physicians/Society of Critical Care Medicine Consensus Conference committee. American College of Chest Physicians/Society of Critical Care Medicine Consensus Conference: definitions for sepsis and organ failure and guidelines for the use innovative therapies in sepsis. Crit Care Med 1992;20:864–74.

7. Esmon CT, Fukudome K, Mather T, et al. Inflammation, sepsis, and coagulation. Haematologica 1999;84:254–9.

8. Rangel-Frausto MS, Pittet D, Costigan M, et al. The natural history of the systemic inflammatory response syndrome (SIRS). A prospective study. JAMA 1995;273: 117–23.

9. Levi M, ten Cate H. Disseminated intravascular coagulation. N Engl J Med 1999;341: 586–92.

10. Gando S, Iba T, Eguchi Y, et al. A multicenter, prospective validation of disseminated intravascular coagulation diagnostic criteria for critically ill patients: comparing current criteria. Crit Care Med 2006;34:625–31.

11. Gando S, Saitoh D, Ogura H, et al. Natural history of disseminated intravascular coagulation diagnosed based on the newly established diagnostic criteria for critically ill patients: results of a multicenter, prospective survey. Crit Care Med 2008;36:145–50.

12. Bakhtiari K, Meijers JC, de Jong E, et al. Prospective validation of the International Society of Thrombosis and Haemostasis scoring system for disseminated intravascular coagulation. Crit Care Med 2004;32:2416–21.

13. Toh CH, Hoots WK, on behalf of the SSC on disseminated intravascular coagulation of the ISTH. The scoring system of the Scientific and Standardization Committee on Disseminated Intravascular Coagulation of the International Society on Thrombosis and Haemostasis: a 5-year overview. J Thromb Haemost 2007;5:604–6.

14. Dempfle CE. Comparing DIC scores: not an easy task indeed. Thromb Res 2009; 124:651–2.

15. Takemitsu T, Wada H, Hatada T, et al. Prospective evaluation of three different diagnostic criteria for disseminated intravascular coagulation. Thromb Haemost 2011;105:40–4.

16. Levi M, Toh CH, Thachil J, et al. Guidelines for the diagnosis and management of disseminated intravascular coagulation. Br J Haematol 2009;145:24–33.

17. Wada H, Asakura H, Okamoto K, et al. Expert consensus for the treatment of disseminated intravascular coagulation in Japan. Thromb Res 2010;125:6–11.

18. Di Nisio M, Baudo F, Cosmi B, et al. Diagnosis and treatment of disseminated intravascular coagulation: Guidelines of the Italian Society for Haemostasis and Thrombosis (SISET). Thromb Res 2012;129(5):e177–e84.

19. Iba T, Asakura H. Comparison between British and Japanese guidelines for the diagnosis and treatment of disseminated intravascular coagulation. Br J Haematol 2010;149:461–2.

20. Levi M. Japanese consensus for disseminated intravascular coagulation (DIC): is it a small world after all? Thromb Res 2010;125:4–5.

21. Gando S. The SISET incorrectly cited the JAAM DIC scoring system. Thromb Res 2012;129:660.

22. Dinarello CA, Gelfand JA, Wolff SM. Anticytokine strategies in the treatment of the systemic inflammatory response syndrome. JAMA 1993;269:1829–35.

23. Nasraway SA. Sepsis research: we must change the course. Crit Care Med 1999;27: 427–30.
24. Levi M, de Jonge E, van der Poll T. New treatment strategies for disseminated intravascular coagulation based on current understanding of the pathophysiology. Ann Med 2004;36:41–9.
25. Gando S, Kameue T, Nanzaki S, et al. Disseminated intravascular coagulation is a frequent complication of systemic inflammatory response syndrome. Thromb Haemost 1996;75:224–8.
26. Siegel T, Seligsohn U, Aghai E, et al. Clinical and laboratory aspects of disseminated intravascular coagulation: a study of 118 cases. Thromb Haemost 1978;39:122–34.
27. Dhainaut JF, Shorr AF, Macias WL, et al. Dynamic evolution of coagulopathy in the first day of severe sepsis: relationship with mortality and organ failure. Crit Care Med 2005;33:341–8.
28. Dhainaut JF, Yan SB, Joyce DE, et al. Treatment effects of drotrecogin alfa (activated) in patients with severe sepsis with or without overt disseminated intravascular coagulation. J Thromb Haemost 2004;2:1924–33.
29. Kienast J, Juers M, Wiedermann CJ, et al. Treatment effects of high-dose antithrombin without concomitant heparin in patients with severe sepsis with or without disseminated intravascular coagulation. J Thromb Haemost 2006;4:90–7.
30. Gando S. Microvascular thrombosis and multiple organ dysfunction syndrome. Crit Care Med 2010;38(Suppl):S35–42.
31. Saito H, Maruyama I, Shimazaki S, et al. Efficacy and safety of recombinant human soluble thrombomodulin (ART-123) in disseminated intravascular coagulation: results of a phase III, randomized, double-blind clinical trial. J Thromb Haemost 2007;5:31–41.
32. Wada H, Wakita Y, Nakase T, et al. Outcome of disseminated intravascular coagulation in relation to the score when treatment begun. Thromb Haemost 1995;74:848–52.
33. Favaloro EJ. Laboratory testing in disseminated intravascular coagulation. Seimin Thromb Haemost 2010;36:458–67.
34. Levi M. DIC: which laboratory tests are most useful. Blood Rev 2011;25:33–7.
35. ten Cate H. Thrombocytopenia: one of the markers of disseminated intravascular coagulation. Pathophysiol Haemost Thromb 2003–2004;33:413–6.
36. Drews RE, Weinberger SE. Thrombocytopenic disorders in critically ill patients. Am J Respir Crit Care Med 2000;162:347–51.
37. Kitchen S, Preston FE. Standardization of prothrombin time for laboratory control of oral anticoagulant therapy. Semin Thromb Hemost 1999;25:17–25.
38. Kim HK, Hong KH, Toh CH, on behalf of the Scientific and Standardization Committee on DIC of the International Society on Thrombosis and Haemostasis. Application of the international normalized ratio in the scoring system for disseminated intravascular coagulation. J Thromb Haemost 2010;8:1116–8.
39. Yu M, Nardella A, Pechet L. Screening tests of disseminated intravascular coagulation: guidelines for rapid and specific laboratory diagnosis. Crit Care Med 2000;28: 1777–80.
40. Franchini M, Di Minno MN, Coppola A. Disseminated intravascular coagulation in hematologic malignancies. Semin Thromb Hemost 2010;36:388–403.
41. Asakura H, Ontachi Y, Mizutani T, et al. An enhanced fibrinolysis prevents the development of multiple organ failure in disseminated intravascular coagulation in spite of much activation of blood coagulation. Crit Care Med 2001;29:1164–8.

42. Madoiwa S, Nunomiya S, Ono T, et al. Plasminogen activator inhibitor 1 promotes a poor prognosis in sepsis-induced disseminated intravascular coagulation. Int J Hematol 2006;84:398–405.
43. Bick RL. Disseminated intravascular coagulation: a review of etiology, pathophysiology, diagnosis, and management: guidelines for care. Clin Appl Thromb Hemost 2002;8:1–31.
44. Wada H, Gabazza E, Nakasaki T, et al. Diagnosis of disseminated intravascular coagulation by hemostatic molecular markers. Semin Thromb Hemost 2000;26:17–21.
45. Asakura H, Wada H, Okamoto K, et al. Evaluation of haemostatic molecular markers for diagnosis of disseminated intravascular coagulation in patients with infections. Thromb Haemost 2006;95:282–7.
46. Kawasugi K, Wada H, Hatada T, et al. Prospective evaluation of haemostatic abnormalities in overt DIC due to various underlying diseases. Thromb Res 2011;128:186–90.
47. Taylor FB, Kinasewiz GT. The diagnosis and management of disseminated intravascular coagulation. Current Hematol Rep 2002;1:34–40.
48. Hoots WK. Non-overt disseminated intravascular coagulation: definition and pathophysiological implications. Blood Rev 2002;16 (Suppl 1):S3–9.
49. Gando S, Wada H, Asakura H, et al. Evaluation of new Japanese diagnostic criteria for disseminated intravascular coagulation in critically ill patients. Clin Appl Thromb Hemost 2005;11:71–6.
50. Gando S, Saitoh D, Ogura H, et al. Disseminated intravascular coagulation (DIC) diagnosed based on the Japanese Association for Acute Medicine criteria is a dependent continuum to overt DIC in patients with sepsis. Thromb Res 2009;123:715–8.
51. Hayakawa M, Gando S, Hoshino H. A prospective comparison of new Japanese criteria versus ISTH criteria. Clin Appl Thromb Hemost 2007;13:172–81.
52. Singh RK, Baronia AK, Sahoo JN, et al. Prospective comparison of new Japanese Association for Acute Medicine (JAAM) DIC and International Society of Thrombosis and Haemostasis (ISTH) DIC score in critically ill septic patients. Thromb Res 2012;129(4):e119–25.
53. Iwai K, Uchino S, Endo A, et al. Prospective external validation of the new scoring system for disseminated intravascular coagulation by Japanese Association for Acute Medicine (JAAM). Thromb Res 2010;126:217–21.
54. Sivula M, Tallgren M, Pettilä V. Modified scorer for disseminated intravascular coagulation in the critically ill. Intensive Care Med 2005;31:1209–14.
55. Volves C, Wuillemin WA, Zeerleder S. International Society on Thrombosis and Haemostasis score for overt disseminated intravascular coagulation predicts organ dysfunction and fatality in sepsis patients. Blood Coagl Fibrinolysis 2006;17:445–51.
56. Cauchie PH, Cauchie CH, Boudjeltia KZ, et al. Diagnosis and prognosis of overt disseminated intravascular coagulation in a general hospital – meaning of the ISTH score system, fibrin monomers, and lipoprotein-C-reactive protein complex formation. Am J Hematol 2006;81:414–9.
57. Angstwurm MW, Dempfle CE, Spannagl M. New disseminated intravascular coagulation score: a useful tool to predict mortality in comparison with Acute Physiology and Chronic Health Evaluation II and Logistic Organ Dysfunction scores. Crit Care Med 2006;34:314–20.
58. Khemani RG, Bart RD, Alonzo TA, et al. Disseminated intravascular coagulation score is associated with mortality for children with shock. Intensive Care Med 2009;35:327–33.

59. Levi M. Disseminated intravascular coagulation in cancer patients. Best Pract Res Clin Haematol 2009;22:129–36.
60. Thachil J, Toh CH. Disseminated intravascular coagulation in obstetric disorders and its acute haematological management. Blood Rev 2009;23:167–76.
61. Dempfle CE, Wurst M, Smolinski M, et al. Use of soluble fibrin antigen instead of D-dimer as fibrin-related marker may enhance the prognostic power of the ISTH overt DIC core. Thromb Haemost 2004;91:812–8.
62. Toh CH, Downey C. Performance and prognostic importance of a new clinical and laboratory scoring system for identify non-overt disseminated intravascular coagulation. Blood Coagl Fibrinolysis 2005;16:69–74.
63. Egi M, Morimatsu H, Wiedermann CJ, et al. Non-overt disseminated intravascular coagulation scoring for critically ill patients: the impact of antithrombin levels. Thromb Haemost 2009;101:696–705.
64. Wada H, Hatada T, Okamoto K, et al. Modified non-overt DIC diagnostic criteria predict the early phase of overt DIC. Am J Hematol 2010;85:691–4.
65. Sawamura A, Hayakawa M, Gando S, et al. Disseminated intravascular coagulation with a fibrinolytic phenotype at an early phase of trauma predicts mortality. Thromb Res 2009;124:608–13.
66. Sawamura A, Hayakawa M, Gando S, et al. Application of the Japanese Association for Acute Medicine disseminated intravascular coagulation diagnostic criteria for patients at an early phase of trauma. Thromb Res 2009;124:706–10.
67. Kobayashi T, Terao T, Maki M, et al. Diagnosis and management of acute obstetrical DIC. Semin Thromb Hemost 2001;27:161–7.
68. Henzan N, Gando S, Uegaki S, et al. Diagnosis of obstetrical disseminated intravascular coagulation (DIC) using newly developed DIC diagnostic criteria for critically ill patients. JJAAM 2007;18:793–802.
69. Yanada M, Matsushihta T, Suzuki M, et al. Disseminated intravascular coagulation in acute leukemia: clinical and laboratory features at presentation. Eur J Haematol 2006;77:282–7.

# Intensive Care Unit Management of Liver-Related Coagulation Disorders

Kevin Dasher, MD, James F. Trotter, MD*

## KEYWORDS

- Coagulopathy • Cirrhosis • International normalized ratio • Liver transplant
- Thrombocytopenia

## KEY POINTS

- Despite exhibiting many hematologic features of coagulopathy, patients with end-stage liver disease may still develop thrombotic complications.
- Thrombocytopenia is a common problem in cirrhotics and is caused primarily by splenomegaly and thrombopoietin deficiency.
- Routine correction of platelet counts is not required before paracentesis and many other procedures.
- Administration of fresh frozen plasma rarely leads to adequate or durable improvement in the prothrombin time.

Coagulopathy, one of the cardinal features of advanced liver disease, is related to multiple factors including impaired synthetic function, thrombocytopenia, excessive fibrinolysis, platelet dysfunction, and disseminated intravascular coagulopathy (DIC). In the intensive care unit (ICU), management of coagulopathy may require treatment, particularly in actively bleeding patients or in preparation for invasive procedures. This article reviews the background of coagulopathy in patients with end-stage liver disease (ESLD) and management options and comments on common clinical scenarios.

## THROMBOCYTOPENIA

Thrombocytopenia occurs in 49% to 64% of patients with end-stage liver disease (ESLD).[1] The most obvious cause of thrombocytopenia in cirrhotic patients is platelet sequestration within an enlarged spleen that is a consequence of portal hypertension.

The authors have nothing to disclose.
Baylor University Medical Center, 3410 Worth Street, Dallas, TX 75246, USA
* Corresponding author.
E-mail address: james.trotter@baylorhealth.edu

Under normal circumstances, one third of an individual's platelets may be sequestered in the spleen. However, with splenomegaly, this number may increase to
90%.[2–4] However, portal decompressive procedures and splenectomy have had an
inconsistent impact on platelet counts.[5] Although splenectomy usually increases
platelet count, approximately 25% of cirrhotic patients will develop postoperative
portal vein thrombosis.[6] Consequently, splenectomy, as a treatment for thrombocytopenia in cirrhosis, is generally discouraged and should be applied only in special
situations.[7]

Another cause of thrombocytopenia in patients with liver disease relates to
thrombopoietin (TPO). Constitutively produced in the liver, TPO is a hormone that
regulates platelet production by stimulating the maturation and proliferation of
megakaryocytes in the bone marrow. In the initial stages of liver disease, when
hepatic function is preserved, TPO production may be normal. However, with the
progression of hepatic failure, TPO levels decrease leading to a reduction in platelet
production and thrombocytopenia.[5] Liver transplantation restores TPO production
and partially corrects the thrombocytopenia associated with cirrhosis.[8]

There is some evidence suggesting that immune-mediated platelet destruction
may make a minor contribute to the thrombocytopenia of liver disease.[9] Feistauer and
colleagues reported that 40% of patients with primary biliary cirrhosis (PBC) have
platelet antibodies targeted against surface glycoproteins GPIb/IX and GPIIb/IIa.
However, only one fourth of PBC patients with these antibodies were thrombocytopenic.[10] Improvement in platelet count after immunosuppressive therapy in these
patients further supports the role of immune-mediated platelet destruction.[11,12]

### Platelet Dysfunction

Besides a reduction in platelet count, defects in qualitative platelet function may also
contribute to the hemostatic defect noted in liver disease. Multiple studies have
shown that template bleeding times correlate with the degree of liver dysfunction.[13]
The bleeding time may be prolonged regardless of platelet count, as impaired platelet
aggregation is also present.[14] Additional factors include a platelet storage pool
defect[15]; defective platelet signal transduction[16]; decreased levels of thromboxane $A_2$
production by platelets; and increased production of endothelial derived growth
factors, nitric oxide, and prostacylin, which may contribute to defective platelet
activation.[17] However, recent studies suggest that compensatory mechanisms may
overcome the defects in platelet hemostasis previously identified in liver patients.
Lisman and colleagues found that platelet aggregation and adhesion to collagen or
fibrinogen is normal in patients with cirrhosis compared to controls.[18] In addition,
Tripodi reported that patients with cirrhosis generate as much thrombin from their
platelets as patients without liver disease.[19]

### IMPAIRED SYNTHESIS OF CLOTTING FACTORS

The liver synthesizes all clotting factors, with the exception of von Willebrand factor
(vWF), tissue plasminogen activator, and plasminogen activator inhibitor type I
(PAI-1), which are derived from endothelial cells.[20] The extent of coagulation
abnormality depends upon the degree of liver impairment.[21] Vitamin K deficiency may
also contribute to impaired hepatic production of clotting factors, although the effect
seems modest. Absorption of fat-soluble vitamins A, D, E, and K requires bile
production. With chronic liver disease, especially in cases with cholestasis, patients
have an increased risk for vitamin K deficiency. Oral cephalosporins and malnutrition
of alcoholism may also predispose to vitamin K deficiency.[22] However, fewer than
10% of patients with cholestatic liver disease (primary biliary cirrhosis) are vitamin K

deficient.[23] Patients with acute liver dysfunction have vitamin K deficiency rates approaching 30%.[24] Although measured levels may be low in liver patients, there is little correlation with prolongation of prothrombin time.[25] Therefore, correction of vitamin K with oral or parenteral supplementation is rarely indicated in the setting of chronic liver disease. However, in patients with acute or subacute fulminant hepatic failure, marked elevations in prothrombin time may improve with vitamin K repletion. Parenteral repletion is more reliable in this setting because bile production (the initial cause of the deficiency) may prevent adequate absorption after oral administration.

## DISSEMINATED INTRAVASCULAR COAGULATION

Disseminated intravascular coagulation describes a syndrome characterized by widespread intravascular coagulation induced by procoagulants in the blood that overcome natural anticoagulant mechanisms. The clinical sequelae of DIC include both clinically evident bleeding from the skin and mucosal surface as well as thrombosis, the combination of which may lead to end-organ damage and death. The characteristic hematologic features include a low platelet count, prolonged prothrombin time, prolonged thrombin time, prolonged partial thromboplastin time, decreased fibrinogen level, and elevated levels of fibrinogen degradation products indicating increased fibrinolytic activity. These same parameters exist in patients with liver disease, raising the question of whether DIC is a frequent component of the coagulopathy of cirrhosis. However, given the stable platelet counts, preserved thrombin generation, high factor VIII levels, and absence of end-organ damage, patients with chronic liver disease do not fulfill classic criteria of DIC.

Given the hematologic profiles of these patients, with features of both DIC and hyperfibrinolysis, the term "accelerated intravascular coagulation and fibrinolysis (AICF)" has been proposed for this group.[26] This term attempts to unify the features of hyperfibrinolysis and DIC present in these patients.

## RISK OF THROMBOSIS

Despite exhibiting many hematologic features of coagulopathy, patients with ESLD may still develop thrombotic complications. In fact, previous studies have demonstrated that patients with liver disease are more prone to the development of venous thromboses.[27] In a population-based study, Sogaard and colleagues reported a relative risk of thromboembolic disease of 1.74 in cirrhotic patients. Similarly, Northup and colleagues found that 0.5% of cirrhotic patients admitted to their facility developed deep venous thrombosis or pulmonary embolus despite laboratory parameters consistent with coagulopathy.[28] In addition, portal venous thrombosis is a common complication in patients with ESLD.[29] The cause of thromboses in liver patients, whose hematologic profile would suggest coagulopathy, is not clear. However, there is some evidence suggesting that there is "rebalancing" of the coagulation system in cirrhotic patients. That is, while thrombocytopenia, impaired platelet function, and prolonged prothrombin time reflect a hemostatic defect involving impaired fibrin clot formation ("coagulopathy") and platelet-mediated primary hemostasis, these parameters are countered by several factors. First, patients with cirrhosis have markedly elevated levels of von Willebrand factor (vWF).[30] These patients also have reduced levels of the metalloprotease that cleaves vWF (ADAMTS13).[31] vWF complexes with factor VIII, a potent generator of thrombin, and protects it from degradation. In addition, levels of the vitamin K–dependent natural anticoagulants protein C and S are decreased in liver disease. The net effect of these changes is a rebalanced coagulation system that may actually favor thrombosis that may occur in the peripheral or portal veins or the arterial system.[32]

## MANAGEMENT OF COAGULOPATHY

The coagulopathy of cirrhosis frequently requires management in the ICU. The two most common scenarios are patients with overt bleeding (usually from the gastrointestinal tract) and in preparation for invasive procedures. Correction of coagulopathy may include platelet transfusion, administration of plasma, cryoprecipitate, or administration of pharmacologic agents.

### Platelet Transfusion

The guidelines for administration of platelets are based primarily on clinical experience and are quite variable. For patients with active bleeding and profound thrombocytopenia, platelet transfusion is indicated. However, the platelet count at which transfusions should be administered depends on the clinical scenario and, in particular, the severity of bleeding. In general, patients requiring transfusion of red blood cells and a platelet count less than 30,000 should be considered for platelet transfusion. For stable thrombocytopenic patients (without evidence of bleeding), empiric platelet transfusions are not indicated, although some intensivists may feel compelled to do so. It is important to remember that the effects of platelet transfusion are limited and short lived. Transfusion of one unit of platelet concentrate will increase platelet count by only 5000 to 10,000 per microliter; the usual dose is one platelet concentrate unit per 10 kg body weight. The response of platelet transfusion may last for only a few hours up to 24 to 48 hours depending on the clinical setting and volume of platelet concentrate transfused. The magnitude of response is frequently blunted by splenomegaly. Other adverse outcomes may include an increase in intravascular volume, risk of alloimmunization, and acquisition of infectious agents.[5]

For invasive procedures, the recommendations for platelet transfusion vary by specialty and type of procedure. For most procedures, platelet counts should be 50,000 or greater per microliter, although some major procedures may have a higher threshold.[33] For percutaneous liver biopsy, there is no increased risk of complications if platelet counts are less than 60,000.[34] A platelet count of 50,000 is recommend for transjugular liver biopsy.[35] Current hepatology practice guidelines state that routine correction of prolonged prothrombin time or thrombocytopenia is not required for paracentesis, although interventional radiology guidelines still call for correction of the platelet count to 50,000.[36]

### Thrombopoietin-Based Agents

The recognition that patients with cirrhosis have reduced levels of TPO suggested that administration of recombinant TPO may have a therapeutic benefit. Two agents, full-length glycosylated recombinant human TPO and polyethylene glycol conjugated megakaryocyte growth factor, have both been studied and found to increase platelet counts in patients with chronic idiopathic thrombocytopenia and chemotherapy-induced thrombocytopenia. The use of these agents was later suspended in the United States after the observation that neutralizing antibodies, resulting in prolonged thrombocytopenia, could develop after TPO administration.[5]

Eltrombopag, an oral thrombopoietin receptor agonist, has been evaluated in the treatment of myelodysplastic syndrome, chronic idiopathic thrombocytopenic purpura, and cirrhotic patients undergoing therapy for hepatitis C. Thrombocytopenia is a common problem in cirrhosis and is exacerbated during treatment of hepatitis C with interferon. Within the hepatitis C virus (HCV) therapy study, patients with HCV cirrhosis were treated with varying doses of eltrombopag to improve the platelet count. Starting platelet counts ranged from 20,000 to 70,000 per microliter. After 4 weeks of treatment with the novel agent, eltrombopag successfully alleviated thrombocytopenia, with an increase in platelet count to greater than 100,000 in up to 95% of patients.[37] However, eltrombopag is currently not approved for use in patients with chronic liver disease and thrombocytopenia given its risk of complications including cataracts and portal venous thrombosis.[38] In addition, portal vein thrombosis has also been reported with the use of romiplostim, a second type of (subcutaneously administered) thrombopoietin receptor agonist.[39]

### Recombinant Activated Factor VII

Recombinant activated factor VII has approval from the US Food and Drug Administration (FDA) for promoting hemostasis in hemophila, particularly those patients with inhibitors of factor VIII and IX. However, current off-label use, which accounts for 97% of total use, includes the management of bleeding in trauma, intracerebral bleeding, and liver dysfunction.[40] Administration of factor VII improves the prothrombin time in nonbleeding cirrhotic patients in a dose-dependent manner.[41] Several formal studies have evaluated the role of factor VII in the control of bleeding during variceal hemorrhage, liver transplantation, and partial hepatectomy. None of these reports demonstrated efficacy of factor VII on the composite endpoint of failure to control bleeding within 24 hours, failure to prevent clinically significant rebleeding or death within 5 days of first dosing. However, subanalyses demonstrate significant changes in the composite endpoint within upper gastrointestinal hemorrhage in patients with Child-Turcotte-Pugh class B and C cirrhosis,[42] higher survival,[43] and reduced transfusion requirements at the time of transplant.[44] In the transplantation study, patients who received factor VII required two fewer units of packed red blood cells, which is clinically trivial given the cost of the drug (see below). The major concern regarding the off-label use of the drug stems from a reported incidence of arterial thrombosis in up to 10% of patients in a pooled analysis.[45] An additional consideration is cost. When given at a dose of 100 $\mu$g/kg, the cost of one dose of factor VII is approximately $7000.[5] Despite FDA warnings for off-label use, there may be a role for factor VII in unique situations such as the requirement for rapid reversal of a profoundly coagulopathic liver patient in need of a medically urgent procedure with a substantial bleeding risk such as heart catheterization or placement of an intracerebral pressure monitor. This benefit must be weighed against risk of thrombosis inherent to ESLD. In addition, the clinician must also be aware that although recombinant factor VIIa infusions may shorten a prolonged prothrombin time, it will not correct the hyperfibrinolysis or platelet dysfunction often noted in patients with liver disease.

### Fresh Frozen Plasma

The most common means to correct an elevated international normalized ratio (INR) is fresh frozen plasma (FFP) infusion. FFP contains all coagulation proteins and inhibitors present in the bloodstream. The use of FFP to correct coagulopathy makes two assumptions: first, that an elevated INR reflects increased risk of bleeding and second, that FFP transfusions will correct the coagulopathy.[46] Within the setting of liver related coagulopathy, an early study demonstrated large infusion (3–9 units) of FFP may not result in correction of prothrombin time and that the effect was short lived.[47,48] In addition, careful analysis has shown that administration of FFP rarely leads to adequate improvement in the prothromin time. Administration of 2 to 4 units of FFP led to adequate correction of the prothrombin time (to <3 seconds over control) in only 10% of cases.[49] Collectively, these studies demonstrate that plasma lacks efficacy in treating bleeding or as prophylaxis for invasive procedures in patients with an INR less than 2. Similar to a platelet infusion, FFP infusion may result in volume overload, transmission of infection, or transfusion reactions. Currently, there is no indication for correction of INR for primary prophylaxis of bleeding. In the setting of active bleeding or prior to invasive procedures, correction of INR to 2 is generally recommended, although the efficacy of this practice is uncertain.

### Desmopressin

Desmopressin (1-deamino-8-D-arginine vasopressin), a synthetic analogue of arginine vasopressin, is used to correct the bleeding time in von Willebrand's disease (vWd) because it increases concentration of vWF in approximately 80% of patients with vWd. It is also used in hemophilia A as it increases concentrations of factor VIII. Initial studies of desmopressin in compensated cirrhosis showed that it shortened the bleeding time and partial thromboplastin time with increases in factor VIII and vWF.[50] In patients undergoing hepatectomy, desmopressin did not reduce intraoperative blood loss despite increases in factor VIII and vWF.[51] In patients with variceal hemorrhage, the combination of desmopressin and terlipressin increased the re-bleeding rate compared with terlipressin alone.[52] Therefore, it is not routinely used in management of patients with ESLD.

### Other Agents

Cryoprecipitate is a fraction of plasma rich in fibrinogen, factor VIII, vWF, and factor XIII. The most common indication for its use is hypofibrinogenemia in the setting of massive hemorrhage. A recent review on this blood product concluded, "despite 45 years of the use of this product, we still have a lot to learn regarding the optimal use of cryoprecipitate."[53(p177)] It has not been explicitly studied in patients with liver disease.

As mentioned previously, vitamin K deficiency is infrequent in patients with liver disease. Nonetheless, a brief course of vitamin K will exclude its deficiency as a contributing factor. Given the unreliable nature of oral vitamin K absorption, one intravenous dose of 10 mg vitamin K is recommended in patients with acute or subacute liver failure with marked elevation in prothrombin time. The mixed micellar K1 formulation has been shown to have a lower risk of anaphylaxis, with no events recorded in among 13 million patients included in post-marketing surveillance.[54]

### PRACTICAL CONSIDERATIONS

The preceding paragraphs have elaborated the abnormal hemostasis parameters in patients with liver disease and various formulations that address these parameters. Subsequent paragraphs explore how these abnormal parameters and therapeutic options should be applied in contemporary practice, with special consideration given to the new paradigm of a "rebalanced" procoagulation/anticoagulation system.

Although coagulopathy is a defining feature of liver disease, there is limited evidence supporting a link between abnormal tests of hemostasis and increased clinical bleeding. No correlation was found between the duration of bleeding from a laparoscopic liver biopsy site and conventional coagulation parameters of prothrombin time, platelet count, or whole blood clot time.[55,56] Early studies also did not demonstrate a link between variceal hemorrhage and impaired hemostasis.[57,58] There are growing data to support a restrictive transfusion policy at the time of liver transplant, irrespective of measured coagulation parameters. These centers report average transfusion requirements of less than 1 unit of packed cells.[59] Collectively, these data indicate that abnormal tests of hemostasis do not markedly impact the rate of clinically significant bleeding in these patients.

Additional causative factors that may explain their bleeding tendency include hemodynamic alterations due to portal hypertension, endothelial dysfunction, endogenous heparin-like substances from bacterial infections, and renal failure.[26] This theory, that factors other than hypocoagulability are responsible for bleeding tendency, has been supported by recognition of normal thrombin generation and enhanced platelet adhesion in patients with cirrhosis.[19] Comparable measures of profibrinolytic and antifibrinolytic activity and vWF have also been documented in cirrhotic patients compared to normal controls.[30,60]

Despite contrary data, the management of bleeding in the patient with liver disease continues to be governed by the dogma of correction of coagulopathy. This frequently entails giving plasma before invasive procedures, platelet infusion in response to arbitrary platelet thresholds, avoidance of deep venous thrombosis prophylaxis given assumption of "auto-anticoagulation," or the use of various expensive ancillary agents without demonstrable clinical benefit. Recent studies have shown that the coagulation system in these patients is rebalanced due to a parallel reduction in both procoagulant and anticoagulant factors. This finite balance is subject to the slightest perturbation, which may result in familiar complications of bleeding or thrombosis. Applying this emerging concept of rebalancing to the care of the individual patient remains an area for future study. At present, recognition of the distinction between abnormal coagulation parameters and bleeding tendency will enhance the care of the patient with chronic liver disease.

## REFERENCES

1. Bashour FN, Teran JC, Mullen KD. Prevalence of peripheral blood cytopenias (hypersplenism) in patients with nonalcoholic chronic liver disease. Am J Gastroenterol 2000;95:2936–9.
2. Aster RH. Pooling of platelets in the spleen: role in the pathogenesis of "hypersplenic" thrombocytopenia. J Clin Invest 1966;45:645–57.
3. Stein SF, Harker LA. Kinetic and functional studies of platelets, fibrinogen, and plasminogen in patients with hepatic cirrhosis. J Lab Clin Med 1982;99:217–30.
4. Harker LA, Finch CA. Thrombokinetics in man. J Clin Invest 1969;48:963–74.
5. Trotter JF. Coagulation abnormalities in patients who have liver disease. Clin Liver Dis 2006;10:665–78, x–xi.
6. Kinjo N, Kawanaka H, Akahoshi T, et al. Risk factors for portal venous thrombosis after splenectomy in patients with cirrhosis and portal hypertension. Br J Surg 2010;97: 910–6.
7. Hayashi PH, Mehia C, Joachim Reimers H, et al. Splenectomy for thrombocytopenia in patients with hepatitis C cirrhosis. J Clin Gastroenterol 2006;40:740–4.
8. Kujovich JL. Hemostatic defects in end stage liver disease. Crit Care Clin 2005;21: 563–87.
9. Bassendine MF, Collins JD, Stephenson J, et al. Platelet associated immunoglobulins in primary biliary cirrhosis: a cause of thrombocytopenia? Gut 1985;26:1074–9.
10. Feistauer SM, Penner E, Mayr WR, et al. Target platelet antigens of autoantibodies in patients with primary biliary cirrhosis. Hepatology 1997;25:1343–5.
11. Pockros PJ, Duchini A, McMillan R, et al. Immune thrombocytopenic purpura in patients with chronic hepatitis C virus infection. Am J Gastroenterol 2002;97:2040–5.
12. Ramos-Casals M, Garcia-Carrasco M, Lopez-Medrano F, et al. Severe autoimmune cytopenias in treatment-naive hepatitis C virus infection: clinical description of 35 cases. Medicine (Baltimore) 2003;82:87–96.

13. Violi F, Leo R, Vezza E, et al. Bleeding time in patients with cirrhosis: relation with degree of liver failure and clotting abnormalities. C.A.L.C. Group. Coagulation Abnormalities in Cirrhosis Study Group. J Hepatol 1994;20:531–6.

14. Escolar G, Cases A, Vinas M, et al. Evaluation of acquired platelet dysfunctions in uremic and cirrhotic patients using the platelet function analyzer (PFA-100): influence of hematocrit elevation. Haematologica 1999;84:614–9.

15. Laffi G, Marra F, Gresele P, et al. Evidence for a storage pool defect in platelets from cirrhotic patients with defective aggregation. Gastroenterology 1992;103:641–6.

16. Laffi G, Marra F, Failli P, et al. Defective signal transduction in platelets from cirrhotics is associated with increased cyclic nucleotides. Gastroenterology 1993;105:148–56.

17. Lisman T, Leebeek FW. Hemostatic alterations in liver disease: a review on pathophysiology, clinical consequences, and treatment. Dig Surg 2007;24:250–8.

18. Lisman T, Adelmeijer J, de Groot PG, et al. No evidence for an intrinsic platelet defect in patients with liver cirrhosis—studies under flow conditions. J Thromb Haemost 2006;4:2070–2.

19. Tripodi A, Salerno F, Chantarangkul V, et al. Evidence of normal thrombin generation in cirrhosis despite abnormal conventional coagulation tests. Hepatology 2005;41: 553–8.

20. Ben-Ari Z, Osman E, Hutton RA, et al. Disseminated intravascular coagulation in liver cirrhosis: fact or fiction? Am J Gastroenterol 1999;94:2977–82.

21. Mammen EF. Coagulation abnormalities in liver disease. Hematol Oncol Clin North Am 1992;6:1247–57.

22. Amitrano L, Guardascione MA, Brancaccio V, et al. Coagulation disorders in liver disease. Semin Liver Dis 2002;22:83–96.

23. Phillips JR, Angulo P, Petterson T, et al. Fat-soluble vitamin levels in patients with primary biliary cirrhosis. Am J Gastroenterol 2001;96:2745–50.

24. Pereira SP, Rowbotham D, Fitt S, et al. Pharmacokinetics and efficacy of oral versus intravenous mixed-micellar phylloquinone (vitamin K1) in severe acute liver disease. J Hepatol 2005;42:365–70.

25. Kowdley KV, Emond MJ, Sadowski JA, et al. Plasma vitamin K1 level is decreased in primary biliary cirrhosis. Am J Gastroenterol 1997;92:2059–61.

26. Caldwell SH, Hoffman M, Lisman T, et al. Coagulation disorders and hemostasis in liver disease: pathophysiology and critical assessment of current management. Hepatology 2006;44:1039–46.

27. Sogaard KK, Horvath-Puho E, Gronbaek H, et al. Risk of venous thromboembolism in patients with liver disease: a nationwide population-based case-control study. Am J Gastroenterol 2009;104:96–101.

28. Northup PG, McMahon MM, Ruhl AP, et al. Coagulopathy does not fully protect hospitalized cirrhosis patients from peripheral venous thromboembolism. Am J Gastroenterol 2006;101:1524–8 [quiz: 1680].

29. Tsochatzis EA, Senzolo M, Germani G, et al. Systematic review: portal vein thrombosis in cirrhosis. Aliment Pharmacol Ther 2010;31:366–74.

30. Lisman T, Bongers TN, Adelmeijer J, et al. Elevated levels of von Willebrand factor in cirrhosis support platelet adhesion despite reduced functional capacity. Hepatology 2006;44:53–61.

31. Mannucci PM, Canciani MT, Forza I, et al. Changes in health and disease of the metalloprotease that cleaves von Willebrand factor. Blood 2001;98:2730–5.

32. Tripodi A, Mannucci PM. The coagulopathy of chronic liver disease. N Engl J Med 2011;365:147–56.

33. Marwaha N, Sharma RR. Consensus and controversies in platelet transfusion. Transfus Apher Sci 2009;41:127–33.

34. Seeff LB, Everson GT, Morgan TR, et al. Complication rate of percutaneous liver biopsies among persons with advanced chronic liver disease in the HALT-C trial. Clin Gastroenterol Hepatol 2010;8:877–83.
35. Malloy PC, Grassi CJ, Kundu S, et al. Consensus guidelines for periprocedural management of coagulation status and hemostasis risk in percutaneous image-guided interventions. J Vasc Interv Radiol 2009;20:S240–9.
36. Grabau CM, Crago SF, Hoff LK, et al. Performance standards for therapeutic abdominal paracentesis. Hepatology 2004;40:484–8.
37. McHutchison JG, Dusheiko G, Shiffman ML, et al. Eltrombopag for thrombocytopenia in patients with cirrhosis associated with hepatitis C. N Engl J Med 2007;357:2227–36.
38. Eltrombopag to reduce the need for platelet transfusion in subjects with chronic liver disease and thrombocytopenia undergoing Elective Invasive Procedures (ELEVATE). GlaxoSmithKline. Available at: http://www.clinicaltrials.gov/ct2/show/NCT00678587?term=NCT00678587&rank=1. Accessed April 18, 2012.
39. Dultz G, Kronenberger B, Azizi A, et al. Portal vein thrombosis as complication of romiplostim treatment in a cirrhotic patient with hepatitis C-associated immune thrombocytopenic purpura. J Hepatol 2011;55:229–32.
40. Logan AC, Yank V, Stafford RS. Off-label use of recombinant factor VIIa in U.S. hospitals: analysis of hospital records. Ann Intern Med 2011;154:516–22.
41. Bernstein DE, Jeffers L, Erhardtsen E, et al. Recombinant factor VIIa corrects prothrombin time in cirrhotic patients: a preliminary study. Gastroenterology 1997;113:1930–7.
42. Bosch J, Thabut D, Bendtsen F, et al. Recombinant factor VIIa for upper gastrointestinal bleeding in patients with cirrhosis: a randomized, double-blind trial. Gastroenterology 2004;127:1123–30.
43. Bosch J, Thabut D, Albillos A, et al. Recombinant factor VIIa for variceal bleeding in patients with advanced cirrhosis: a randomized, controlled trial. Hepatology 2008;47:1604–14.
44. Lodge JP, Jonas S, Jones RM, et al. Efficacy and safety of repeated perioperative doses of recombinant factor VIIa in liver transplantation. Liver Transpl 2005;11:973–9.
45. Levi M, Levy JH, Andersen HF, et al. Safety of recombinant activated factor VII in randomized clinical trials. N Engl J Med 2010;363:1791–800.
46. Abdel-Wahab OI, Healy B, Dzik WH. Effect of fresh-frozen plasma transfusion on prothrombin time and bleeding in patients with mild coagulation abnormalities. Transfusion 2006;46:1279–85.
47. Spector I, Corn M, Ticktin HE. Effect of plasma transfusions on the prothrombin time and clotting factors in liver disease. N Engl J Med 1966;275:1032–7.
48. Williamson LM, Llewelyn CA, Fisher NC, et al. A randomized trial of solvent/detergent-treated and standard fresh-frozen plasma in the coagulopathy of liver disease and liver transplantation. Transfusion 1999;39:1227–34.
49. Youssef WI, Salazar F, Dasarathy S, et al. Role of fresh frozen plasma infusion in correction of coagulopathy of chronic liver disease: a dual phase study. Am J Gastroenterol 2003;98:1391–4.
50. Burroughs AK, Matthews K, Qadiri M, et al. Desmopressin and bleeding time in patients with cirrhosis. Br Med J (Clin Res Ed) 1985;291:1377–81.
51. Wong AY, Irwin MG, Hui TW, et al. Desmopressin does not decrease blood loss and transfusion requirements in patients undergoing hepatectomy. Can J Anaesth 2003; 50:14–20.
52. de Franchis R, Arcidiacono PG, Carpinelli L, et al. Randomized controlled trial of desmopressin plus terlipressin vs. terlipressin alone for the treatment of acute variceal hemorrhage in cirrhotic patients: a multicenter, double-blind study. New Italian Endoscopic Club. Hepatology 1993;18:1102–7.

53. Callum JL, Karkouti K, Lin Y. Cryoprecipitate: the current state of knowledge. Transfus Med Rev 2009;23:177–88.
54. Pereira SP, Williams R. Adverse events associated with vitamin K1: results of a worldwide postmarketing surveillance programme. Pharmacoepidemiol Drug Saf 1998;7:173–82.
55. Ewe K. Bleeding after liver biopsy does not correlate with indices of peripheral coagulation. Dig Dis Sci 1981;26:388–93.
56. Dillon JF, Simpson KJ, Hayes PC. Liver biopsy bleeding time: an unpredictable event. J Gastroenterol Hepatol 1994;9:269–71.
57. Boks AL, Brommer EJ, Schalm SW, et al. Hemostasis and fibrinolysis in severe liver failure and their relation to hemorrhage. Hepatology 1986;6:79–86.
58. Basili S, Ferro D, Leo R, et al. Bleeding time does not predict gastrointestinal bleeding in patients with cirrhosis. The CALC Group. Coagulation Abnormalities in Liver Cirrhosis. J Hepatol 1996;24:574–80.
59. Massicotte L, Beaulieu D, Thibeault L, et al. Coagulation defects do not predict blood product requirements during liver transplantation. Transplantation 2008;85:956–62.
60. Lisman T, Leebeek FW, Mosnier LO, et al. Thrombin-activatable fibrinolysis inhibitor deficiency in cirrhosis is not associated with increased plasma fibrinolysis. Gastroenterology 2001;121:131–9.

# Etiology and Significance of Thrombocytopenia in Critically Ill Patients

Robert I. Parker, MD

## KEYWORDS

- Platelets • Thrombocytopenia • Heparin-induced thrombocytopenia • Critically ill
- Intensive care unit

## KEY POINTS

- The development or worsening of thrombocytopenia following ICU admission is an indicator of poor prognostic risk.
- Scoring systems for HIT are best at identifying those patients at low risk for HIT.
- Over diagnosis of HIT results in increased hospital length of stay, cost and morbidity. Platelet injury assays are best at identifying those patients who have HIT as a consequence warrant a change in anticoagulant therapy.
- Drugs frequently employed in critically-ill patients are a common cause of thrombocytopenia in the ICU.
- Sepsis can cause thrombocytopenia by increased platelet destruction and/or decreased platelet production.

## INTRODUCTION

Thrombocytopenia is a common occurrence in intensive care unit (ICU) patients, with incidence rates ranging from 13% to nearly 60% in recent published series.[1–5] Although there is some variability in the incidence of thrombocytopenia based on ICU and patient demographics (less in pediatric and surgical patients when compared to adults and medical ICU patients), published reports encompass patients from diverse parts of the world and in all types of ICUs and describe a truly universal occurrence. Although many of these critically ill patients will demonstrate thrombocytopenia on admission to the ICU, for the vast majority, thrombocytopenia is not the primary cause, or even a substantial cause, for that admission. However, of those patients

The author has nothing to disclose.
Department of Pediatrics, Stony Brook University School of Medicine, Pediatric Hematology/Oncology, Stony Brook Long Island Children's Hospital, HSC T-11, Room 029, 100 Nicolls Road, Stony Brook, NY 11794–8111, USA
*E-mail address:* Robert.Parker@stonybrookmedicine.edu

Crit Care Clin 28 (2012) 399–411
http://dx.doi.org/10.1016/j.ccc.2012.04.007
0749-0704/12/$ – see front matter © 2012 Elsevier Inc. All rights reserved.

criticalcare.theclinics.com

**Table 1**
**Causes of thrombocytopenia**

| Decreased Production | Increased Destruction (Clearance) |
|---|---|
| ➢ Primary marrow failure or disorder<br>• Fanconi anemia<br>• Congenital amegakaryocytic Thrombocytopenia<br>• Thrombocytopenia and absent radii [TAR] syndrome<br>• Myelodysplastic disorders | ➢ Nonimmune<br>• Mechanical (intravascular devices)<br>  ○ IABP, PA, CVL catheters<br>• Microangiopathic<br>  ○ TTP, DIC, SBE, vasculitis<br>  ○ Drugs<br>• Splenic pooling<br>  ○ Passive (eg, splenomegaly secondary to liver disease)<br>  ○ Active (hypersplenism)<br>• Platelet aggregation<br>  ○ Drugs |
| ➢ Secondary marrow failure (suppression)<br>• Severe idiopathic aplastic Anemia<br>• Severe malnutrition<br>• Sepsis<br>• Drugs (eg, penicillins, cephalosporins, vancomycin, anticonvulsants, H2 blockers) | ➢ Immune<br>• Platelet-specific antibodies (ie, ITP)<br>• Immune complex (eg, autoimmune disorders)<br>• Cell-mediated (eg, hypersplenism, hemophagocytic syndrome/macrophage activation syndrome)<br>• PTP<br>• Sepsis |
| ➢ Infiltrative diseases of the marrow<br>• Neoplastic<br>  ○ Acute leukemia<br>  ○ Widespread marrow metastases<br>• Non-neoplastic<br>  ○ Storage disorders (eg, Gaucher disease) | ➢ Immune: Drugs<br>• Multiple drugs have been shown to cause immune-mediated thrombocytopenia including antiepileptics (eg, valproic acid), gold compounds, thiazides, quinine/quinidine, vancomycin. |
| ➢ Iatrogenic (anticipated consequence of therapy)<br>• Chemotherapy<br>• Radiation therapy<br>  ○ External radiation<br>  ○ Internal radiation | ➢ Immune: HIT<br>• HIT antibodies are most commonly associated with exposure to unfractionated heparin but can also be induced after exposure to low molecular weight heparins, antifactor Xa agents, and danaparoid. |

*Abbreviations:* CVL, central venous catheters; IABP, intra-aortic balloon pump; PA, pulmonary artery; SBE, subacute bacterial endocarditis.

who do not exhibit thrombocytopenia at the time of ICU admission, many will develop thrombocytopenia while in the ICU.[5] Although thrombocytopenia clearly increases the risk for bleeding, both spontaneous and resulting from invasive procedures, and results in higher mortality and greater morbidity in ICU patients,[4] the presence of thrombocytopenia may also alert intensivists to possible underlying causes for their patients' critical illness, or to developing complications resulting from their treatment. Consequently, an understanding of the possible causes and clinical significance of thrombocytopenia is essential to good ICU care.

## CAUSES AND RISK FACTORS FOR THROMBOCYTOPENIA IN THE ICU

The causes of thrombocytopenia can be divided into essentially two categories: decreased production or increased destruction (loss). **Table 1** presents a partial listing of the clinical conditions frequently resulting in thrombocytopenia in critically ill patients, and a framework of how to think about these possible causes. Although there may be some overlap in conditions producing both marrow suppression of thrombopoiesis and increased destruction of platelets, and there are multiple sub-categories under each major group, dividing the causes into conditions that result in increased platelet destruction and those that cause decreased platelet production provides a convenient starting point for clinical and laboratory evaluation. At times, the clinical scenario may give clues as to the cause of thrombocytopenia. These clues include degree of thrombocytopenia, drug history, underlying medical conditions, pre-illness platelet count, and time course of the development of thrombocytopenia, to name a few.[6,7] The time course of thrombocytopenia at times may give the clinician a clue to its origin; a rapid marked decrease occurring 1 to 2 weeks after a drug initiation or a surgical procedure is suggestive of an immune-mediated process whereas a gradual decline is more suggestive of marrow suppression of thrombo-poiesis or possible subacute platelet consumption.[7]

Several studies have attempted to define associated risk factors for the develop-ment of thrombocytopenia in the ICU.[3–5,8–12] Not surprisingly, drug exposure, most notably unfractionated heparin, intravascular devices (eg, central venous catheters, pulmonary artery catheters, intra-aortic balloon pumps), and higher severity of illness score on ICU admission have all been reported to represent factors associated with an increased risk of thrombocytopenia during an ICU stay. Sepsis developing during an ICU admission has specifically been noted to be associated with the development of thrombocytopenia.

## PROGNOSTIC SIGNIFICANCE OF THROMBOCYTOPENIA DEVELOPING DURING ICU ADMISSION

Multiple studies have shown that the development of thrombocytopenia during an ICU admission is associated with increased length of stay, morbidity, and mort-ality.[3,5,10,13–20] This association has been noted in both medical and surgical patients, in pediatric and adult patients, and is particularly apparent as a prognostic indicator in sepsis.[16–19] In aggregate, these studies demonstrate an increased mortality in patients who develop thrombocytopenia (generally defined as a platelet count less than 150,000/$\mu$L or a greater than 30%–50% decrease from ICU admission platelet count) after ICU admission compared to those whose platelet count remained stable or recovered within the first week of ICU stay.[4,14,16] In addition, patients whose thrombocytopenia worsened or persisted beyond the first 4 to 7 days of ICU admission exhibited an even greater risk of mortality.[13–18] Some studies have shown a decreased risk of mortality in patients whose platelet counts recovered during their ICU admission, and increased risk of mortality with more severe and/or prolonged thrombocytopenia.[4,14,16,20] As these patients were critically ill and generally exhibited significant clinical abnormalities in addition to thrombocytopenia, one can reasonably ask if the thrombocytopenia was directly associated with mortality. On multivariate analysis, the association of thrombocytopenia with mortality continues to be demon-strated. Consequently, it is not unreasonable to conclude that the development or persistence of thrombocytopenia in ICU patients may identify patients who have critical illness that carries with it a risk of mortality that is greater than that of the "typical" ICU patient.

Although severe thrombocytopenia increases the incidence and risk of bleeding, either spontaneously or in association with trauma, procedures, or critical illness,[13,17] the cause of excess mortality in thrombocytopenic ICU patients is generally not due to uncontrolled bleeding resulting from a low platelet count. Consequently, one must look for a related, though secondary, reason for the demonstrated association of thrombocytopenia with mortality. Indeed, in a recent analysis of intraventricular hemorrhage (IVH) and thrombocytopenia in neonates, the increased incidence of IVH in neonates with thrombocytopenia was not dependent on the degree of thrombocytopenia observed.[21] This observation suggests that it may be the process causing thrombocytopenia rather than the thrombocytopenia itself that is of paramount importance. Data developed over the past several years have elucidated the myriad interconnections of hemostasis and the immune response, many of which occur at the level of the endothelium and involve platelet–endothelial cell interactions[22] (this excellent review contains a broader discussion of this topic). Many of these points of interaction involve the inflammatory response and may explain why thrombocytopenia frequently accompanies illnesses characterized by marked, often poorly regulated, inflammatory responses.[23] With this as a background, it is not surprising that the development of thrombocytopenia in ICU patients is associated with the multiorgan failure and frequently precedes the development of organ dysfunction.[10,13,15,17] Our greater, and developing, understanding of the role platelets play in inflammation may potentially help to identify new targets for treating these disorders.

## DISORDERS ASSOCIATED WITH INCREASED PLATELET DESTRUCTION
### *Immune-Mediated Platelet Destruction*

Immune (antibody)-mediated platelet destruction can be primary (ie, idiopathic [immune] thrombocytopenia [ITP]), secondary to an underlying immune-mediated illness (eg, systemic lupus erythematosus [SLE]) with immune complex binding via platelet $F_c$ receptors, or the consequence of drug exposure (including heparins, anticonvulsants [eg, valproic acid], gold compounds, cephalosporin class antibiotics, and quinidine, to name some of the more common causative drugs).

### *Heparin-Induced Thrombocytopenia*

Whereas the paradigm for immune platelet destruction outside of the ICU may be idiopathic (immune) thrombocytopenia (ITP), in the ICU, heparin-induced thrombocytopenia (HIT) is more frequently considered and potentially of greater concern because of the increased risk for thrombosis accompanying this disorder. HIT results from the production of antibodies directed toward a heparin–platelet factor IV complex formed when heparin binds to the platelet surface.[22,24,25] These antibodies not only result in macrophage-mediated clearance of antibody-coated platelets from the circulation, but by binding to platelet $F_c\gamma IIa$ receptors, they result in platelet activation, thereby producing a prothrombotic phenotype. A similar process activating endothelial cells has been hypothesized, with some data supporting this hypothesis recently being reported.[26] Treatment of HIT requires removal of all heparin exposure from the patient (including heparin flushes and heparin-coated catheters) and the initiation of alternate modes of anticoagulation (eg, direct thrombin inhibitors). The reader is referred to several well written and comprehensive reviews on this topic.[25,27–30] Left unaddressed, or in the presence of platelet transfusions to ostensibly correct the thrombocytopenia, often catastrophic thrombosis may occur.

### *Diagnosis of HIT*

To assist in the diagnosis of HIT, clinical scoring algorithms have been developed.[22,31–33] The most widely employed is the so-called "4 T's": (1) **T**hrombocytopenia, (2) **T**iming (of thrombocytopenia), (3) **T**hrombosis, and (4) other causes for **T**hrombocytopenia (**Table 2**). Although the presence of a low 4T score consistently

| Table 2 | |
|---|---|
| **The 4T scoring system for heparin-induced thrombocytopenia** | |
| **Thrombocytopenia:** Development of thrombocytopenia with a >50% decrease in platelet count after exposure to heparin. This drop does not require that the platelet count fall below 140,000–150,000/μL (the usual lower limit of normal for platelet count). Severe thrombocytopenia (<10,000/μL) is rarely caused by HIT. | **2 points:** Decrease in platelets >50% previous value, **or** lowest platelet count is 20,000–100,000/μL. <br> **1 point:** Decrease in platelet count 30%–50% of prior value, **or** lowest platelet count is <10,000/μL. <br> **0 points:** If decrease in platelets is <30% from prior value, **or** lowest platelet count is <10,000/μL. |
| **Timing:** Drop in platelet count occurring between the 5th and 10th day after heparin exposure if the patient had not been exposed to heparin previously. The decrease in platelets may be evident earlier if patient had been exposed to heparin recently (ie, within 100 days). | **2 points:** Decrease in platelets occurs 5–10 days after first heparin exposure, **or** decrease occurs within 1 day of reexposure to heparin (if prior heparin exposure within 30 days). <br> **1 point:** Decrease in platelets occurs after 10 days from first heparin exposure **or** decrease occurs within 1 day of reexposure to heparin (if prior heparin exposure within 30–100 d). <br> **0 points:** If decrease in platelets is earlier than 5 days but patient had no prior heparin exposure. |
| **Thrombosis:** Is there any evidence for thrombotic events since initiating heparin exposure? This may be overt thrombosis such as DVT or may be more subtle, taking the form of microvascular thrombi causing renal insufficiency, hypoxemia, altered mental status, acrocyanosis or other clinical findings suggestive of vascular occlusion. Events that occur shortly after a platelet infusion are particularly suspicious. | **2 points:** New proven thrombosis, skin necrosis, or systemic reaction. <br> **1 point:** Progressive or recurrent thrombosis, silent thrombosis, or red skin lesions. <br> **0 points:** No symptoms. |
| **Other causes of thrombocytopenia:** A diagnosis of HIT can be made only if there are no other potential causes for thrombocytopenia present. Such causes include sepsis with or without evidence of microangiopathy. | **2 points:** No other cause for thrombocytopenia identified. <br> **1 point:** Possible alternative cause present. <br> **0 points:** Definite alternative cause present. |

A score of 0–8 points is possible. A score of 0–3 indicates HIT is unlikely: no change in anticoagulant therapy indicated. A score of 4–5 indicates intermediate probability of HIT: depending on the clinical setting and physician judgment, alternate anticoagulant therapy may be considered while more sensitive and specific tests for HIT are obtained. A score of 6–8 is highly suggestive of HIT; alternate anticoagulant therapy should be considered while more sensitive and specific tests for HIT are obtained.

identifies those patients unlikely to have HIT, multiple studies have shown that an intermediate or high score is less useful in predicting results of laboratory testing obtained to confirm a HIT diagnosis. Consequently, other such screening tools have been developed but none has been widely employed or studied (such as The **H**IT **E**xpert **P**robability [HEP] Score[33]). At this time, a platelet injury assay such as the serotonin release assay (SRA) is considered the "gold standard" for the diagnosis of HIT. Some laboratories utilize heparin-induced platelet aggregation to confirm a diagnosis of HIT, but this test does not appear to be as specific for true HIT as is the

SRA. However, because each of these assays are time and labor intensive and require fresh platelets and, in the case of the SRA radiolabeled serotonin, they are of limited usefulness in "real time" clinical decision making. As a result, enzyme-linked immonosorbent assay (ELISA)- based assays to detect heparin-dependent anti-PF4 antibodies are generally employed in the diagnosis of HIT. However, these assays have been found to overdiagnose HIT because they are not specific for platelet-activating heparin-dependent anti-PF4 antibodies.[34–36] Consequently, these assays have a moderate-to-high negative predictive value but a low positive predictive value (as does the 4T scoring system). Patients who are shown to have very high titer antibodies, however, have been shown to be more likely to have platelet-activating antibodies.[37–39] Based on this finding, some investigators have recommended raising the discriminate optical density reading (OD) for the ELISA assays to improve the positive predictive value of the tests. Because of the poor performance of the currently available ELISA assays in identifying patients most likely to have HIT, new assays to identify the presence of platelet-activating antibodies, or to identify the presence of activated platelets in circulation have been developed.[40–43] Although promising, none of these tests has yet gained wide clinical implementation.

### Treatment of suspected or confirmed HIT
Once a diagnosis of HIT is made or suspected, all heparin exposure, including heparin flushes and heparin-bonded catheters, must be removed. Patients on heparin for therapeutic anticoagulation require continued anticoagulation with an alternate agent. In addition, patients in whom HIT has been diagnosed who require a surgical procedure, must be treated by a different perioperative algorithm and their surgery is frequently delayed. Many of these patients are cardiac surgery patients who are at high risk already. Platelet transfusions are contraindicated in HIT due to the high risk of initiating a thrombotic event. The risk for thrombosis with HIT (HITT; HIT with thrombosis) persists for up to 30 days after removal of all heparin exposure, with the greatest risk being the 48 to 72 hours before and immediately after the suspected diagnosis. Because of the time required for the establishment of an anticoagulated state with warfarin, vitamin K antagonist therapy is not recommended in the period immediately after removal of heparin exposure. Consequently, any patient with suspected HIT requires anticoagulation with an agent that will effect immediate anticoagulation and is believed to carry a low risk of inducing the development of cross-reacting, heparin-dependent anti-PF4 antibodies. Currently, in the United States, the only agents approved for this indication are the direct thrombin inhibitors (DTIs; argatroban, lepirudin).[44,45] In addition, the activated factor X inhibitor (anti-Xa) fondaparinux has also been shown to be effective in preventing thrombosis in HIT. However, as there have been rare cases in which HIT antibodies have been induced by this agent, use of drugs in this class of drug is not recommended as front-line therapy for HIT.[46] Although the heparanoid Danaparoid has been successfully used to treat HIT, this agent is no longer available in the United States.

### Is overdiagnosis of HIT a problem?
Owing to the imprecision in diagnosing HIT, many patients are suspected of having HIT, but the diagnosis is actually confirmed in only a few. However, even when a case of HIT is not confirmed there are modifications required in patient management. As a consequence of the need for prolonged anticoagulation, patients diagnosed with, or labeled as having, HIT incur significant added medical costs owing to extended length of hospital stay (frequently within the ICU) and the costs of alternate, expensive

anticoagulant therapy. Recent analyses have placed the additional burden at $163,396 to greater than $1 million per quality adjusted life year (QALY; 2004 US$) depending on the test and treatment strategy employed.[47] Other economic analyses place the hospital cost at $14,000 to $20,000 per suspected HIT case without taking into account decreased bed utilization costs. Economic analyses performed in other health care systems demonstrated similar, though not identical, increase in costs associated with each suspected HIT case.[48–50]

### Non-HIT Immune Thrombocytopenia

Other causes of immune-mediated thrombocytopenia include ITP (primary and secondary), drugs and post-transfusion purpura (PTP).[51,52] In primary immune thrombocytopenia, formerly referred to as idiopathic thrombocytopenic purpura, antibodies are produced that are directed against specific antigens on the platelet surface. Epitopes on glycoprotein IIb/IIIa are the most commonly identified targets for these antibodies, owing at least in part to the fact that this is the most numerous and dense antigenic structure on the platelet. The antiplatelet GPIIb/IIIa drug abciximab (Reopro) has been shown to produce acute and delayed (up to 12 days after exposure) immune thrombocytopenia.[53,54] Secondary immune thrombocytopenia results from the binding of immune complexes to the platelet surface via $F_c$ receptors, from the binding of drug–antibody complexes to the platelet, or binding of antibodies to a neoantigen created by a platelet–drug complex created on the platelet surface. Sepsis has been associated with an immune thrombocytopenia due to immune complex binding to the platelet. Treatment of primary immune thrombocytopenia frequently involves corticosteroids, intravenous-immunoglobulin G (IV-IgG) or IV anti-RhD antibody. Treatment for secondary immune thrombocytopenia depends on the related condition: immunosuppression for thrombocytopenia occurring as a component of a global immune-mediated illness (eg, systemic lupus erythematosus), removal of offending drug if drug related, or treatment of the source of infection if sepsis related. In some cases, immune thrombocytopenia may result from activation of cell-mediated immunity without antibody production.

PTP is a poorly understood clinical complex in which a patient, usually a multiparous woman or a previously transfused male, develops an immune thrombocytopenia after transfusion with platelets or other blood product containing platelets or platelet particles (ie, whole blood, packed red blood cells [pRBCs], leukocytes, and fresh frozen plasma [FFP]). Most affected individuals have platelets that are negative for the human platelet antigen 1a (HPA-1a; formerly PL^A1).[55,56] Although the initial immune reaction is directed against the donor platelets, this triggers production of alloantibodies directed against autologous platelets. The exact mechanism whereby transfused platelets trigger the production of alloantibodies is not clear. PTP develops 5 to 12 days after transfusion and is potentially life threatening. The disorder is generally self limited, but IV-IgG is the treatment of choice for severe or persistent thrombocytopenia. In refractory cases plasmapheresis may be required. There are also reports of successful management of critical bleeding using PL^A1-negative platelets.[57] However, as alloantibodies causing PTP can be directed against other platelet specific epitopes, this treatment cannot be assumed to be uniformly effective. In some cases, PTP has been misdiagnosed as HIT.[58]

### Nonimmune Thrombocytopenia

The most common causes of nonimmune platelet destruction fall under the category of microangiopathic processes. Included in this group are disseminated intravascular coagulation (DIC), thrombotic thrombocytopenic purpura (TTP), and hemolytic uremic syndrome (HUS). In addition, a localized consumption of platelets can occur with mechanical heart valves or other intravascular devices (eg, aortic balloon pumps, left ventricular assist devices and infected heart valves subacute bacterial endocarditis). Each of these disorders is characterized by some degree of hemolysis, as indicated by the presence of schistiocytes on peripheral blood smear. DIC is primarily a thrombotic disorder with secondary hemorrhage resulting from uncontrolled consumption of platelets and clotting factors.[59,60] Myriad conditions can initiate this process including sepsis, hemolysis, trauma/crush injury, obstetric mishaps, and vasculitis. In general, the treatment of choice is to treat the underlying condition initiating the process. TTP is a microangiopathic process in which thrombocytopenia and microvascular thrombosis are the most prominent features.[61] The classic presentation consists of a pentad of features (thrombocytopenia, microangiopathic hemolytic anemia, fever, mental status changes, and renal insufficiency), although most patients do not present with all five elements. Thrombocytopenia and microangiopathic hemolytic anemia are most consistently noted on presentation. Most cases have been shown to result from either a congenital or acquired (antibody-mediated) deficiency of the von Willebrand factor cleaving metalloprotease ADAMTS13.[61] Associated inciting events include pregnancy, human immunodeficiency virus (HIV) infection, and some drugs (eg, ticlopidine, cyclophosphamide).[62,63] Plasma exchange via plasmapheresis is the treatment of choice, although simple plasma infusions have also been shown to be effective in early/mild cases.[64,65] Although aspirin is frequently a component of therapeutic regimens, its effectiveness has not been validated. Platelet transfusions are not contraindicated, but they should be used with caution because of a concern of inducing microvascular platelet deposition. HUS is a pathophysiologically related disorder in that it is characterized by microvascular thrombosis with microangiopathic hemolytic anemia, thrombocytopenia, renal insufficiency, and altered mental status. However, unlike TTP, deficiency of ADAMTS13 has not been causally implicated and hemolytic anemia and renal insufficiency are the prominent clinical features. In the United States, HUS most commonly results from endothelial cell injury caused by a verotoxin produced by a pathogenic strain of *Escherichia coli* (O157:H7) or by *Shigella* strains elaborating shigatoxin.[61,65] Treatment of HUS is largely supportive, but may require dialysis.[66] Platelet transfusion is generally not required owing to the relatively mild degree of thrombocytopenia. Of interest, the complement-directed monoclonal antibody eculizumab has been shown to prevent the need for dialysis in a single case report of atypical HUS in an adult.[67]

## THROMBOCYTOPENIA SECONDARY TO DECREASED PRODUCTION OF PLATELETS

Thrombocytopenia resulting from decreased marrow production of platelets may be secondary to a congenital marrow failure syndrome (eg, Fanconi anemia, congenital amegakaryocytic thrombocytopenia, thrombocytopenia, and absent radii syndrome [TAR]), or result from acquired causes[68–70] (see **Table 1**). While Fanconi anemia is slowly progressive and frequently does not produce significant cytopenias until later in life, both TAR and congenital amegakaryocytic thrombocytopenia present in infancy. Myelodysplastic syndromes may be considered under either the congenital or acquired categories of marrow failure depending on the nature of the disorder. With the exception of the congenital transient myelodysplastic disorder associated with Down syndrome (trisomy-21), these disorders tend to present in older adults, though earlier presentations are possible. Myelodyspasia can be the consequence of prior cancer chemotherapy and may develop following hematopoietic stem cell transplantation. Severe idiopathic aplastic anemia is an acquired marrow aplasia thought to represent an immune-mediated process directed against hematopoietic stem cells.[71,72] This is generally thought to follow a viral illness. Patients who do not have an appropriate matched-related hematopoietic stem cell donor are treated with intensive immunosuppression. From the majority of causes of productive thrombocytopenia, the patient will be thrombocytopenic before ICU admission and the thrombocytopenia per se is not the cause for the admission.

Within the ICU, sepsis and drugs are the most common causes of productive thrombocytopenia that develops while in the ICU, with up to 25% of ICU patients developing drug-induced thrombocytopenia.[1,3,5–8,10] Multiple drugs have been implicated in thrombocytopenia, and it is often difficult to pinpoint the exact drug causing the thrombocytopenia, as ICU patients may frequently be receiving multiple drugs that could potentially reduce platelet count. However, multiple antibiotics (vancomycin, penicillins, cephalosporins), H2 blockers (cimetidine, ranitidine), and anticonvulsants (valproicacid, phenytoin) have commonly been implicated.[1,3,5,6] In the absence of a microangiopathic/consumptive process, a slow and steady decline in platelets, and a nadir platelet count below 20,000/$\mu$L is generally more suggestive of drug-induced thrombocytopenia resulting from marrow suppression. A rapid decline occurring over 1 to 2 days is more suggestive of an immune mechanism (drug or non–drug-related), while a consumptive coagulopathy may manifest a variable rate in platelet decline depending on the aggressiveness of the process.[7] When a drug-related cause for thrombocytopenia is suspected, the treatment of choice is to remove further exposure to the drug. In the case of suppression of platelet production, platelet counts should start to show recovery within 5 to 7 days but generally not before 48 hours.

## SUMMARY

Thrombocytopenia is common in ICU patients, and its presence predicts increased morbidity, mortality, and hospital resource utilization. When thrombocytopenia develops or worsens after ICU admission, this is associated with a worsening of the underlying process, causing the patient's platelet count to be decreased on admission, or indicates that there is a new process ongoing. In either event, the clinician must be aware of the myriad causes for decreasing platelets and initiate appropriate investigations even if the patient is not actively bleeding. Drugs, consumptive coagulopathy (eg, DIC) and heparin-induced thrombocytopenia should all be on the clinician's radar, although HIT is still a relatively infrequent occurrence. However, because of the often catastrophic consequences of not identifying HIT, this disorder must be considered whenever a patient exposed to heparin develops thrombocytopenia.

## REFERENCES

1. Priziola JL, Smythe MA, Dager WE. Drug-induced thrombocytopenia in critically ill patients. Crit Care Med 2010;38(6 Suppl):S145–54.
2. Hanes SD, Quarled DA, Boucher BA. Incidence and risk factors of thrombocytopenia in critically ill trauma patients. Ann Pharmacother 1997;31:285–9.
3. Cawley MJ, Wittbrodt ET, Boyce EG, et al. Potential risk factors associated with thrombocytopenia in a surgical intensive care unit. Pharmacotherapy 1999;19:108–13.
4. Strauss R, Wehler M, Mehler K, et al. Thrombocytopenia in patients in the medical intensive care unit: bleeding prevalence, transfusion requirements and outcome. Crit Care Med 2002;30:1765–71.
5. Hui P, Cook DJ, Lim W, et al. The frequency and clinical significance of thrombocytopenia complicating critical illness: a systematic review. Chest 2011;139:271–8.
6. Wazny LD, Ariano RE. Evaluation and management of drug-induced thrombocytopenia in the acutely ill patient. Pharmacotherapy 2000;20:292–307.

7. Greinacher A, Selleng K. Thrombocytopenia in the intensive care unit patient. Hematology Am Soc Hematol Educ Program 2010;2010:135–43.

8. Bonfiglio MF, Traeger SM, Kier KL, et al. Thrombocytopenia in intensive care patients: a comprehensive analysis of risk factors in 314 patients. Ann Pharmacother 1995;29: 835–42.

9. Shalansky SJ, Verma AK, Levine M, et al. Risk markers for thrombocytopenia in critically ill patients: a prospective analysis. Pharmacotherapy 2002;22:803–13.

10. Sharma B, Sharma M, Majumder M, et al. Thrombocytopenia in septic shock patients—a prospective observational study of incidence, risk factors and correlation with clinical outcome. Anaesth Intensive Care 2007;35:874–80.

11. Vicente Rull JR, Loza Aguirre J, de la Puerta E, et al. Thrombocytopenia induced by pulmonary artery flotation catheters: a prospective study. Intensive Care Med 1984; 10:29–31.

12. Vonderheide RH, Thadhani R, Kuter DJ. Association of thrombocytopenia with the use of intra-aortic balloon pumps. Am J Med 1998;105:27–32.

13. Vanderschueren S, De Weerdt A, Malbrain M, et al. Thrombocytopenia and prognosis in intensive care. Crit Care Med 2000;28:1871–6.

14. Akca S, Haji-Michael P, de Mendonca A, et al. Time course of platelet counts in critically ill patients. Crit Care Med 2002;30:753–6.

15. Morerau D, Timsit JF, Vesin A, et al. Platelet count decline: an early prognostic marker in critically ill patients with prolonged ICU stays. Chest 2007;131:1735–41.

16. Krishnan J, Morrison W, Simone S, et al. Implications of thrombocytopenia and platelet course on pediatric intensive care unit outcomes. Pediatr Crit Care Med 2008;9:502–5.

17. Nydam TL, Kashuk JL, Moore EE, et al. Refractory postinjury thrombocytopenia is associated with multiple organ failure and adverse outcomes. J Trauma 2011;70: 401–6.

18. Masrouki S, Mebazaa MS, Mestiri T, et al. Risk factors of mortality in critically ill patients with thrombocytopenia. Ann Fr Anesth Reanim 2004;23:783–7.

19. Vandijck DM, Blot SI, De Waele JJ, et al. Thrombocytopenia and outcome in critically ill patients with bloodstream infection. Heart Lung 2010;39:21–6.

20. Olmez I, Zafar M, Shahid M, et al. Analysis of significant decrease in platelet count and thrombocytopenia, graded according to NCI-CTC, as prognostic risk markers for mortality and morbidity. J Pediatr Hematol Oncol 2011;33:585–8.

21. Von Lindern JS, van den Bruele T, Lopriore E, et al. Thrombocytopenia in neonates and the risk of intraventricular hemorrhage: a retrospective cohort study. BMC Pediatr 2011;11:16.

22. Warkentin TE, Aird WC, Rand JH. Platelet-endothelial interactions: sepsis, HIT, and antiphospholipid syndrome. Hematology Am Soc Hematol Educ Program 2003; 2003:497–519.

23. Katz JN, Kolappa KP, Becker RC. Beyond thrombosis: the versatile platelet in critical illness. Chest 2011;139:658–68.

24. Poncz M. Mechanistic basis of heparin-induced thrombocytopenia. Semin Thorac Cardiovasc Surg 2005;17:73–9.

25. Warkentin TE. Heparin-induced thrombocytopenia in critically ill patients. Crit Care Clin 2011;27:805–23.

26. Davidson SJ, Wadham P, Rogers L, et al. Endothelial cell damage in heparin-induced thrombocytopenia. Blood Coagul Fibrinolysis 2007;18:317–20.

27. Greinacher A, Farner B, Kroll H, et al. Clinical features of heparin-induced thrombocytopenia including risk factors for thrombosis: a retrospective analysis of 408 patients. Throb Haemost 2005;94:132–5.

28. Selleng K, Warkentin TE, Greinacher A. Heparin-induced thrombocytopenia in intensive care patients. Crit Care Med 2007;35:1165–76.

29. Warkentin TE, Greinacher A, Koster A, et al; American College of Chest Physicians. Treatment and prevention of heparin-induced thrombocytopenia; 8th ed: American College of Chest Physicians evidence-based clinical practice guidelines. Chest 2008; 133(6 Suppl):340S–380S.

30. Kato S, Takahashi K, Ayabe K, et al. Heparin-induced thrombocytopenia: analysis of risk factors in medical inpatients. Br J Haematol 2011;154:373–7.

31. Lo GK, Juhl D, Warkentin TE, et al. Evaluation of pretest score (4 T's) for the diagnosis of heparin-induced thrombocytopenia in two clinical settings. J Thromb haemost 2006;4:759–65.

32. Crowther MA, Cook DJ, Albert M, et al; The Canadian Critical Care Trials Group. The 4Ts scoring system for heparin-induced thrombocytopenia in medical-surgical intensive care unit patients. J Crit Care 2010;25:287–93.

33. Cuker A, Arepally G, Crowther MA, et al. The HIT Expert Probability (HEP) Score: a novel pre-test probability model for heparin-induced thrombocytopenia based on broad expert opinion. J Thromb Haemost 2010;8:2642–50.

34. Verma AK, Levine M, Shalansky SJ, et al. Frequency of heparin-induced thrombocytopenia in critical care patients. Pharmacotherapy 2003;23:745–53.

35. Juhl D, Eichler P, Lubenow N, et al. Incidence and clinical significance of anti-PF4/heparin antibodies of the IgG, IgM, and IgA class in 755 consecutive patient samples referred for diagnostic testing for heparin-induced thrombocytopenia. Eur J Haematol 2006;76:420–6.

36. Greinacher A, Juhl D, Strobel U, et al. Heparin-induced thrombocytopenia: a prospective study on the incidence, platelet-activating capacity and clinical significance of antiplatelet factor 4/heparin antibodies of the IgG, IgM, and IgA classes. J Thromb Haemost 2007;5:1666–73.

37. Warkentin TE, Sheppard JL, Moore JC, et al. Quantitative interpretation of optical density measurements using PF4-dependent enzyme-immunoassays. J Thormb Haemost 2008;6:1304–12.

38. Ruf KM, Bensadoun ES, Davis GA, et al. A clinical-laboratory algorithm incorporating optical density value to predict heparin-induced thrombocytopenia. Thromb Haemost 2011;105:553–9.

39. Baroletti S, Hurwitz S, Conti NA, et al. Thrombosis in suspected heparin-induced thrombocytopenia occurs more often with high antibody levels. Am J Med 2012;125: 44–9.

40. Pouplard C, Leroux D, Regina S, et al. Effectiveness of a new immunoassay for the diagnosis of heparin-induced thrombocytopenia and improved specificity when detecting IgG antibodies. Thromb Haemost 2010;103:145–50.

41. Bakchoul T, Giptner A, Bein G, et al. Performance characteristics of two commercially available IgG-specific immunoassays in the assessment of heparin-induced thrombocytopenia (HIT). Thromb Res 2011;127:345–8.

42. Morel-Kopp MC, Tan CW, Brighton TA, et al; on behalf of the ASTH Clinical Trials Group. Validation of whole blood impedance aggregometry as a new diagnostic tool for HIT. Results of a large Australian study. Thromb Haemost 2012;107(3):575–83.

43. Prechel MM, Escalante V, Drenth AF, et al. A colorimetric, metabolic dye reduction assay detects highly activated platelets: application in the diagnosis of heparin-induced thrombocytopenia. Platelets 2012;23:69–80.

44. Warkentin TE. Agents for the treatment of heparin-induced thrombocytopenia. Hematol Oncol Clin North Am 2010;24:755–75.

45. Hassell K. Heparin-induced thrombocytopenia: diagnosis and management. Thromb Res 2008;123(Suppl 1):S16–21.
46. Warkentin TE, Pai M, Sheppard JL, et al. Fondaparinux treatment of acute heparin-induced thrombocytopenia confirmed by the serotonin-release assay; a 30-month, 16-patient case series. J Thromb Haemost 2011;9:2389–96.
47. Patrick AR, Winkelmayer WC, Avorn J, et al. Strategies for the management of suspected heparin-induced thrombocytopenia: a cost-effectiveness analysis. Pharmacoeconomics 2007;25:949–61.
48. Smythe MA, Koerber JM, Fitzgerald M, et al. The financial impact of heparin-induced thrombocytopenia. Chest 2008;134:568–73.
49. Elalamy I, Le Gal G, Nachit-Ouinekh F, et al. Heparin-induced thrombocytopenia: an estimate of the average cost in the hospital setting in France. Clin Appl Thromb Hemost 2009;15:428–34.
50. Nanwa N, Mittmann N, Knowles S, et al. The direct medical costs associated with suspected heparin-induced thrombocytopenia. Pharmacoeconomics 2011;29:511–20.
51. Liebman H. Other immune thrombocytopenias. Semin Hematol 2007;44(4 Suppl 5):S24–34.
52. Cines DB, Liebman H, Stasi R. Pathobiology of secondary immune thrombocytopenia. Semin Hematol 2009;46(1 Suppl 2):S2–14.
53. Lajus S, Clofent-Sanchez G, Jais C, et al. Thrombocytopenia after abciximab use results from different mechanisms. Thromb Haemost 2010;103:651–61.
54. Nurden P, Clofent-Sanchez G, Jais C, et al. Delayed immunologic thrombocytopenia induced by abciximab. Thromb Haemost 2004;92:820–8.
55. Gonzalez CE, Pengetze YM. Post-transfusion purpura. Curr Hematol Rep 2005;4:154–9.
56. Shtalrid M, Shvidel L, Vorst E, et al. Post-transfusion purpura: a challenging diagnosis. Isr Med Assoc J 2006;8:672–4.
57. Loren AW, Abrams CS. Efficacy of HPA-1a (PLA1)-negative platelets in a patient with post-transfusion purpura. Am J Hematol 2004;76:2258–62.
58. Lubenow N, Eichler P, Albrecht D, et al. Very low platelet counts in post-transfusion purpura falsely diagnosed as heparin-induced thrombocytopenia: report of four cases and review of literature. Thromb Res 2000;100:115–25.
59. Kitchens CS. Thrombocytopenia and thrombosis in disseminated intravascular coagulation (DIC). Hematology Am Soc Hematol Educ Program 2009:240–6.
60. Ten Cate H. Thrombocytopenia: one of the markers of disseminated intravascular coagulation. Pathophysiol Haemost Thromb 2003;33:413–6.
61. Chapman K, Seldon M, Richards R. Thrombotic microangiopathies, thrombotic thrombocytopenic purpura, and ADAMTS-13. Semin Thromb Hemost 2012;38:47–54.
62. Medina PJ, Sipols, George JN. Drug-associated thrombotic thrombocytopenic purpura-hemolytic uremic syndrome. Curr Opin Hematol 2001;8:286–93.
63. Zakarija A, Kwaan HC, Moake JL, et al. Ticlopidine- and clopidogrel-associated thrombotic thrombocytopenic purpura (TTP): review of clinical, laboratory, epidemiological, and pharmacovigilance findings (1989–2008). Kidney Int Suppl 2009;112:S20–4.
64. Coppo P, Veyradier A. Current management and therapeutical perspectives in thrombotic thrombocytopenic purpura. Presse Med 2012. [Epub ahead of print].
65. Clark WF. Thrombotic microangiopathy: Current knowledge and outcomes with plasma exchange. Semin Dial 2012. [Epub ahead of print].

66. Goldwater PN, Bettelheim KA. Treatment of enterohemorrhagic *E. coli* (EHEC) infection and hemolytic uremic syndrome (HUS). BMC Med 2012;10:12.
67. Ohanian M, Cable C, Halka K. Eculizumab safely reverses neurologic impairment and eliminates need for dialysis in severe atypical hemolytic uremic syndrome. Clin Pharmacol 2011;3:5–12.
68. Tamary H, Alter BP. Current diagnosis of inherited bone marrow failure syndromes. Pediatr Hematol Oncol 2007;24:87–99.
69. Dokal I, Vulliamy T. Inherited aplastic anaemias/bone marrow failure syndromes. Blood Rev 2008;22:141–53.
70. Tamary H, Nishri D, Yacobovich J, et al. Frequency and natural history of inherited bone marrow failure syndromes: the Israeli Inherited Bone Marrow Failure registry. Haematologica 2010;95:1300–7.
71. Keohane EM. Acquired aplastic anemia. Clin Lab Sci 2004;17:165–71.
72. Davies JK, Guinan EC. An update on the management of severe idiopathic aplastic anaemia in children. Br J Haematol 2007;136:549–64.

# A Reappraisal of Plasma, Prothrombin Complex Concentrates, and Recombinant Factor VIIa in Patient Blood Management

Lawrence Tim Goodnough, MD

KEYWORDS

- Plasma • Prothrombin complex concentrates • Recombinant factor VIIa
- Blood management

KEY POINTS

- Understand role of plasma therapy in reversal of warfarin coagulopathy.
- Know the contents, limitations, and risks of prothrombin complex concentrates for treatment of warfarin coagulopathy.
- Know current recommended best practices for emergency reversal of warfarin.

## INTRODUCTION

There are a number of critical care settings in which patients can present with massive and/or refractory hemorrhage and require urgent or emergent therapy, listed in **Box 1**. In trauma-associated bleeding, for example, management problems arise associated with a number of coagulopathies: hemodilution from blood losses replaced with colloid or crystalloid, consumption due to loss of coagulation factors and platelets in clot formation, consumption through disseminated intravascular coagulation (DIC) related to tissue anoxia and microvascular damage, and primary or secondary fibrinolysis related to endothelial damage and/or clot formation. These problems have led to development of massive transfusion protocols with proactive strategies of 1:1:1 replacement of red blood cells, plasma, and platelets for patients with massive hemorrhage such as trauma.[1] Similar approaches have been published for patients with life-threatening postpartum hemorrhage.[2] Laboratory evidence of DIC is also an underlying sequela with refractory bleeding in patients undergoing complex surgeries

Departments of Pathology and Medicine, Stanford University School of Medicine, 300 Pasteur Drive, Room H-1402, 5626, Stanford, CA 94305-5626, USA
E-mail address: ltgoodno@stanford.edu

Crit Care Clin 28 (2012) 413–426
http://dx.doi.org/10.1016/j.ccc.2012.04.002
0749-0704/12/$ – see front matter © 2012 Elsevier Inc. All rights reserved.
criticalcare.theclinics.com

---

**Box 1**
**Some clinical settings with refractory or massive bleeding requiring urgent or emergent therapy**

- Coagulopathy of liver disease: acute fulminant hepatitis or cirrhosis
- Warfarin-associated coagulopathy
- Trauma
- Postpartum
- Complex surgical procedures: liver transplantation, cardiothoracic surgery
- Gastrointestinal lesions: esophageal varices, diverticulosis
- Sepsis with disseminated intravascular coagulation

---

such as liver transplantation or cardiothoracic surgical procedures, as well as in patients with the coagulopathy of liver disease. Moreover, the clinical significance of traditional laboratory assays for evaluation of the hemostatic pathway (prothrombin time and partial thromboplastin) in some settings such as in liver disease is currently undergoing reassessment.[3,4] Finally, strategies in acute reversal of warfarin-associated coagulopathy are undergoing scrutiny regarding the relative role(s) of plasma, prothrombin complex concentrates (PCCs), and recombinant activated factor VII (rFVIIa) therapy to supplement vitamin K administration in the management of these patients. This review summarizes current approaches in utilization of hemostatic agents for management of patients in the critical care setting who have refractory or massive bleeding.

## PLASMA THERAPY

There are a number of plasma products currently licensed and available to the transfusion service: fresh frozen plasma (FFP; plasma frozen within 8 hours of collection), FP24 (plasma frozen within 24 hours of collection), thawed plasma (TP; thawed FFP or FP24 units relabeled with an extended shelf life to 96 hours beyond their previous postthaw shelf life of 24 hours),[5] and liquid plasma (plasma units never frozen, a product with a shelf life of 26 days at 4°C).[6] Plasma products carry known risks (**Box 2**[7–12]): pathogen-causing disease transmission, transfusion-related volume overload, transfusion-related acute lung injury (TRALI), and allergic transfusion

---

**Box 2**
**Some current known risks of plasma therapy**

Pathogens transmissible by blood[7]:

- 1:500,000 (hepatitis B) to 1:2,000,000 (hepatitis C, human immunodeficiency virus)

Allergic transfusion reactions[8]:

- 1%–2% for severe, up to 15% for mild

Transfusion-related volume overload[9]:

- 6% in prospective surveillance studies.

Transfusion-related acute lung injury[10,11,12]:

- Estimated to be 1:5,000–10,000 before risk mitigation policies for female plasma donors; reduced to 1:60,000 in 2006, 1:170,000 in 2008.

reactions are some examples. Plasma products generally are stored at −18°C for up to 1 year, so they must be thawed before issue as well as compatible with the patients documented blood type (ABO/Rh). AABB Standards for Transfusion Services[13,14] mandate policies that reduce the risk of TRALI. As a result, most blood centers now restrict collection of plasma from female donors with past history of pregnancy (a source of leukocyte-reactive, neutrophilic-specific antibodies or human leukocyte antigen antibodies that can cause TRALI).[15] Such policies have substantially reduced the currently recognized incidence of TRALI (see **Box 2**).[12]

Limitation of procurement of plasma to male donors and females who have never been pregnant, however, has imposed inventory constraints that have made availability of FFP impractical for many blood centers. At the authors' institution they provide FP24 units, which are converted to TP upon 24 hours after thawing; they also provide liquid plasma (blood type AB) for emergency-release support of patients with emergent needs for plasma therapy whose blood type is unknown or blood group B or AB.[1,2,16] Because these are cellular (never frozen) products, they are irradiated and are also not regarded as cytomegalovirus-safe ("CMV-safe"). Rh status for liquid plasma is also relevant. These plasma products have been approved by the authors' hospital transfusion committee for use at the discretion of their transfusion service as alternatives to FFP for treatment of coagulopathies, because levels of factor VIII (which is the temperature-labile clotting factor of primary concern) are clinically not relevant outside the treatment of hemophilia A. Because the terminology *FFP* persists both in the literature and at the bedside, FFP is used to denote these other plasma products in this review.

A recent report from the AABB Transfusion Medicine Clinical Practice Committee reviewed published evidence for recommendations in plasma therapy.[17] Outside the setting of trauma, when literature reviewed was limited to level 1 evidence, no survival benefit to plasma therapy was found. A "weak" recommendation was given for reversal of warfarin-associated coagulopathy in medical/surgical emergencies such as intracerebral hemorrhage (ICH), based on the quality of evidence.[18] Nevertheless, the panel believed that the efficacy of plasma outweighed its potential risks (specified in the report as increased occurrence of TRALI and reduced plasma inventory) for patients with ICH and warfarin-associated coagulopathy.

The level of recommendation and the grading of evidence as "low," however, could be in part attributable to two factors: there is a paucity of studies to support that abnormal coagulation test results predict bleeding, particularly in the setting of invasive procedures,[19] and for patients who may need/benefit from plasma therapy, the delayed administration and inadequate dosing strategies reported in the literature have been unable to show convincing evidence for a benefit for plasma therapy.[20,21]

Lack of enthusiasm and logistical/technical barriers (**Table 1**) in this and other settings have led to approaches for plasma therapy that are perhaps too little, too late. First, transfusion services must identify the patient's blood group type before issuing blood type–compatible plasma; for patients unknown to the institution and/or without a historic blood type in the patient record within the past year, considerable time (up to 60 minutes) can elapse from presentation until a blood type can be ordered, drawn, and determined by the transfusion service. Second, because plasma is stored frozen at −18°C, further time (30−45 minutes) may be required to thaw and issue plasma. Third, the volume for each plasma unit infused (approximately 200−250 mL) represents a challenge regarding volume overload, which occurs commonly in an elderly population who may have preexisting comorbidities such as atrial fibrillation/cardiovascular disease. The dosing of plasma needed to correct the coagulopathy has often been underestimated and therefore may be subtherapeutic in some clinical practices;

| Table 1 | |
|---|---|
| **Potential barriers for plasma therapy in patients with intracerebral hemorrhage** | |
| **Barrier** | **Estimated Time Needed** |
| Liquid AB plasma not widely available | |
| Patient blood type must be determined | Up to 60 min |
| Plasma units must be thawed | 30–45 min |
| Plasma volume requires careful management to avoid circulatory overload | 30 min per unit |
| Plasma dosing is underestimated | |

plasma therapy of 15 to 30 mL/kg is necessary to restore hemostatic clotting factor levels to 30% to 50% of normal[21] in acute reversal of warfarin toxicity.

In the coagulopathy of liver disease, plasma therapy may not represent appropriate management.[4] In liver disease, the extent of coagulopathy as measured by the prothrombin time (PT) or international normalized ratio (INR) is not predictive of bleeding complications.[22–24] Thrombin-generation assays[25,26] that measure platelet procoagulant activity have found that patients with cirrhosis have primary hemostasis via cell-mediated pathways that are not measured by traditional laboratory assays such as PT and partial PT (PTT). Increasingly, studies indicate that these patients can undergo major hemostatic challenges such as liver biopsies and surgical procedures without plasma therapy and without bleeding complications.[19] Moreover, normalization of laboratory tests in this setting is rarely achieved by plasma therapy.[27] The most clinically relevant bleeding problems are a consequence of local vascular abnormalities and increased venous pressures.[24,28] Thus, a more conservative plasma therapy approach would be to avoid volume and fluid overload that paradoxically favor hemorrhage, such as portal hypertension and endothelial damage.[3] Alternative therapies to plasma infusion have been proposed to improve hemostasis in patients with liver disease, including the infusion of low volume PCCs or antifibrinolytic agents that lack the side effects of volume overload.[4]

## PROTHROMBIN COMPLEX CONCENTRATES

PCCs are either activated (ie, to allow for bypassing inhibitors to factor VIII or factor IX in the treatment of patients with hemophilia A or B), or are nonactivated: some of these PCCs are approved for use in factor IX deficiency (hemophilia B) and of which some are approved for reversal of warfarin toxicity. These nonactivated PCC products currently available worldwide are listed in **Table 2**.[21] The nonactivated PCCs are further categorized based on the presence (four factor) or absence (three factor) of sufficient levels of factor VII.[29] PCCs that contain all four (including factor VII) of the vitamin K–dependent clotting factors (II, VII, IX, X) are approved in the European Union,[30] vary in other countries such as Canada and Australia, and are not yet approved in the United States. A four-factor PCC product (Beriplex, CSL Behring, King of Prussia, PA, USA)[31] is currently undergoing regulatory review in the United States for emergency reversal of warfarin coagulopathy in patients with major bleeding[31] and also for perioperative management of patients receiving warfarin therapy.[32] Three-factor PCCs are approved in the United States only for the replacement of factor IX. Use of these three-factor PCCs for reversal of warfarin is controversial; although they can be demonstrated to normalize INR,[33] one report showed a suboptimal effect in correcting INR because of minimal increments in levels

**Table 2**
**PCC products**

| Product (Manufacturer) | Factors Levels (IU/mL) | | | |
|---|---|---|---|---|
| | II | VII | IX | X |
| Available in the United States: | | | | |
| PCCs, three-factor (II, IX, X) | | | | |
| Profilnine SD (Grifols)[a] | ≤150 | ≤35 | ≤100 | ≤100 |
| Bebulin VH (Baxter)[a] | 24–38 | <5 | 24–38 | 24–38 |
| Available outside the United States: | | | | |
| PCCs, four-factor (II, VII, IX, X) | | | | |
| Beriplex (CSL Behring)[b] | 20–48 | 10–25 | 20–31 | 22–60 |
| Octaplex (Octapharma)[c] | 14–38 | 9–24 | 25 | 18–30 |
| Cofact (Sanguin)[d] | 14–35 | 7–20 | 25 | 14–35 |
| Prothromplex T (Baxter)[e] | 30 | 25 | 30 | 30 |
| PCCs, three-factor (II, IX, X) | | | | |
| Prothromplex HT (Baxter)[f] | 30 | – | 30 | 130 |

The values given for factor contents are the number of units present per 100 factor IX units in each vial.

[a] Product insert specifies: "Indicated for replacement of Factor IX in patient with hemophilia B. Not indicated for treatment of Factor VII deficiency."

[b] United Kingdom, European Union.

[c] United Kingdom, Canada, European Union.

[d] European Union.

[e] Austria.

[f] Australia.

*From* Goodnough LT, Shander AS. How I treat warfarin-associated coagulopathy in patients with intracerebral hemorrhage. Blood 2011;117:6091–9; with permission.

of factor VII.[29] In contrast, four-factor PCCs are approved outside the United States for replacement of the vitamin K–dependent clotting factors.[34] Reviews focusing on the roles of PCC and other options in reversing warfarin-associated coagulopathy have been recently published.[21,35–38]

Guidelines from a number of medical societies have also been published. Five guidelines (**Table 3**)[39–44] have recommended that PCC can be given as an alternative to FFP in order to increase levels of vitamin K–dependent clotting factors. Two of these guidelines[42] indicate that PCC is the preferred treatment, and one indicates that plasma is not indicated if a four-factor PCC is available.[43] One guideline specifies that if three-factor PCC is administered, FFP should also be given in order to provide replacement of factor VII.[39] One review of emergency reversal of anticoagulation therapy in neurosurgical patients has recommended the concomitant administration of a three-factor concentrate (4000 IU) and rFVIIa (1.0 mg) for patients treated at one trauma center in the United States.[45] Another recent review of PCCs for reversal of warfarin concluded that "PCC should be compared directly in randomized controlled trials [with] other treatment strategies including FFP and rFVIIa, evaluating effect on patient outcomes"[38]; normalization of the INR is just a surrogate end point.[46] This lack of consensus on the role of PCC therapy relative to plasma therapy is in part due to the variability in their contents and clotting factor levels[29,47]; their regulatory approval status in different

**Table 3**
**Published guidelines for reversal of warfarin anticoagulation in patients with intracerebral hemorrhage**

| Society (yr) | Vitamin K (mg) | Plasma (mL/kg) | | PCC (U/kg) | rFVII |
|---|---|---|---|---|---|
| Australian (2004)[39] | IV (5–10 mg) | Yes (NS) | AND | Yes (NS)[a] | NS |
| EU Stroke (2006)[40] | IV (5–10 mg) | Yes (10–40) | OR | Yes (10–50) | NS |
| AHA (2010)[41] | IV (NS) | Yes (10–15) | OR | Yes (NS) | No |
| French (2010)[42] | Oral or IV (10 mg) | Yes (NS)[b] | OR | Preferred (25–50) | No |
| British Standards (2011)[43] | IV (5 mg) | No | | Yes (NS) | No |
| ACCP (2012)[44] | IV (10 mg) | Yes (NS) | OR | Preferred (NS) | Yes[c] |

[a] If a three-factor PCC is administered, FFP is also recommended as a source of factor VII.
[b] Use of plasma only when PCCs not available.
[c] Use of PCCs or rFVIIa may vary depending on availability.
*Abbreviations:* NS, not specified; PCC, prothrombin complex concentrate; rFVIIa, Recombinant Human Activated Factor VII; IV, Intravenous.

countries; their uncertain availability among hospital formularies, particularly in community hospitals; and their potential risks of thrombogenicity.

Product information for activated PCCs such as FEIBA (VH Immuno; Baxter AG, Vienna, Austria) and Autoplex-T (Baxter, Roundtree, IL, USA) state under warnings that they "must be used only for patients with circulating inhibitors to one or more coagulation factors and should not be used for the treatment of bleeding episodes resulting from coagulation factor deficiencies."[48,49] Additionally, as stated in the package inserts, the presence of DIC is a contraindication to their use. Nevertheless, despite the even greater potential risk of thrombogenicity compared with nonactivated PCCs, use of FEIBA has been recommended for reversal of warfarin in life-threatening bleeding if four-factor PCCs are not available.[50] A chart review of 72 patients who received FEIBA for warfarin reversal compared with 69 patients who were treated with FFP in life-threatening bleeding indicated faster and more effective reduction of INR with FEIBA, but similar survival rates and length of hospital stay between the cohorts. However, 7% of the FEIBA-treated patients suffered potentially related adverse events.[50]

The safety of PCCs in the setting of emergency reversal of warfarin anticoagulation remains a subject of debate. A recent prospective study of 173 patients treated with PCC found that 4.6% of patients had a thrombotic event but attributed these adverse events to cessation of anticoagulant therapy for underlying and ongoing risks of thrombosis.[51] A recent study in a pig model of coagulopathy with blunt liver injury found that whereas 35 IU/kg PCC improved coagulation and attenuated blood loss, increased doses (50 IU/kg) of PCC therapy seemed to increase the risk of thromboembolism and DIC.[52] Thrombogenicity has been a recognized problem for patients,[53,54] in part related to the presence of activated clotting factors (for which heparin and antithrombin III have been added to some preparations), and also in part due to presence of other preexisting thromboembolic risk factors that resulted in initiation of warfarin in these patients (eg, venous thrombosis, atrial fibrillation) or new, concurrent risk factors (eg, trauma, head injury).

The authors previously reported a patient who was initially successfully treated with rFVIIa for refractory, massive hemorrhage while on extracorporeal membrane

**Table 4**
**Potential risks and limitations of PCC therapy**

| Product | Risks and Limitations |
|---|---|
| Single-Donor Plasma | Longer time to administer |
| | Volume constraints |
| | Ransmissible disease, known/unknown |
| | llergic reactions |
| | TRALI |
| PCCs | Limited availability |
| | Some preparations lack factor VII |
| | Donor pools: 3000 to 20,000 |
| | Transmissible disease, known/unknown (for nonenveloped pathogens) |
| | Thrombogenicity |

oxygenation post cardiothoracic surgery but suffered massive thrombosis after subsequently receiving an activated PCC.[55] Another case of fatal intracardiac thrombosis following rapid administration of activated PCC for urgent warfarin coagulation reversal has also been reported.[56] Reported incidence of thromboembolic events published between 1998 and 2008 ranged from 0 to 7% (overall weighted mean of 2.3%), with higher and repeated dosing potentially associated with higher risk.[38] Multinational trials on patients receiving a four-factor PCC product at various infusion speeds for urgent vitamin K antagonist reversal have supported the safety and efficacy of rapid infusion of PCC in these patients.[57,58] However, it is noteworthy that one recommendation is, "Whenever possible, patients receiving PCCs should be under low dose heparin prophylaxis,"[47] underscoring that use of PCCs in this setting is accompanied by risks of thrombosis. A recent review[59] of eight clinical studies identified a thromboembolic event rate of .9% associated with PCC therapy. Studies of optimal dosing strategies for PCC, including fixed versus variable (weight-based) dosage, provide a basis for future research.[60]

As pooled blood product derivatives, PCCs also have potential risks of transmitting infectious agents.[61] Various processing methods such as nanofiltration, solvent detergent treatment, and vapor heating have been used to inactivate pathogens in commercially available PCCs and pooled plasma products.[62] The cost-effectiveness of such products with pathogen reduction technology is an area of current debate.[63,64] Potential risks and limitations of PCC therapy compared with plasma therapy are summarized in **Table 4**.

## RECOMBINANT ACTIVATED FACTOR VII

Recombinant FVIIa is thought to act via two mechanisms, both of which serve to restrict coagulation activation to the site of tissue damage (**Fig. 1**).[65] First, rFVIIa complexes directly with tissue factor (TF) released from the subendothelium at sites of vascular disruption. The TF-rFVIIa complex then activates the remainder of the common coagulation cascade via activated factor X. Alternatively, rFVIIa may bind to activated platelets, which also concentrates factor X activation to sites of tissue injury. The factor Xa generated by these two mechanisms ultimately drives the thrombin burst, which cleaves fibrinogen to fibrin, thus initiating the formation of the fibrin meshwork critical to secondary coagulation and clot stabilization. The potential role for rFVIIa in tissue factor-independent clotting has raised concern for its site

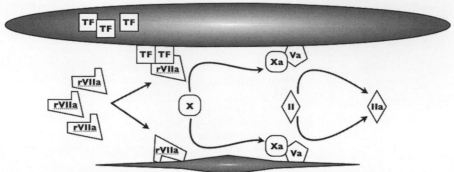

**Fig. 1.** Recombinant human factor VIIa mechanisms of action. At pharmacologic levels, rFVIIa complexes with tissue factor (TF) from the subendothelium and on the surface of cells at the site of tissue damage. rFVIIa also binds to the surface of activated platelets. Factor X (FX) is activated by rFVIIa-TF and rFVIIa on the surface of platelets to FXa, which complexes with FVa to catalyze the conversion of pro-thrombin (FII) to thrombin (FIIa). FII, II; FIIa, IIa; FVa, Va; FXa, Xa. (*Adapted from* Poon MC. Use of recombinant factor VIIa in hereditary bleeding disorders. Curr Opin Hematol 2001;8:312–8; with permission.)

specificity and the risk for off-target thrombosis. Accordingly, the US Food and Drug Administration (FDA) required addition of a black box warning to the package insert in 2005 warning physicians of the risk of thromboembolic complications when the agent is used, in view of these safety concerns for thromboembolic adverse events (TAEs), along with continued uncertainty regarding its level of efficacy.

Approved indications of rFVIIa in the United States and European Union include treatment of bleeding episodes (or prevention of bleeding from invasive procedures) in patients with congenital hemophilia A or B with inhibitors to factors VIII or IX, patients with congenital factor VII deficiency, and in patients with acquired hemophilia. Additionally, it is approved for patients with an inherited qualitative platelet defect in treatment of Glanzmann thrombasthenia in the European Union. However, these approved indications accounted for only 3121 (4.2%) of 73,747 cases reported to use rFVIIa in the United States from 2000 to 2008,[66] and off-label use of rFVIIa in a variety of other clinical settings has continued to rise rapidly (**Fig. 2**). For example, use of rFVIIa in patients not on warfarin who had spontaneous ICH increased eightfold, from 250 cases in 2004 to 2010 cases in 2008, accounting for 11% of all off-label rFVIIa usage. Other off-label categories include cardiovascular surgery and trauma in an attempt to address uncontrolled hemorrhage in these settings. Finally, early reports of the off-label use of rFVIIa in the successful management of warfarin-associated ICH in patients with refractory bleeding led to development of policies for oversight of its off-label use.[67] A subsequent systematic literature review found only limited available evidence for five off-label indications that suggested no mortality reduction with rFVIIa use.[68]

Case reports have described the successful use of rFVIIa in patients with warfarin-associated anticoagulation and ICH,[69–71] and studies have indicated that doses of 15 to 20 $\mu$gm/kg rFVIIa can normalize INR values when used to treat warfarin-associated deficiencies of functional vitamin K–dependent clotting factors.[72] Nonetheless, concerns have been raised whether the effect goes beyond mere

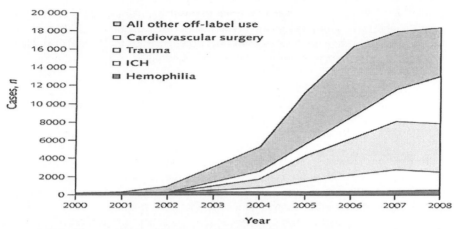

**Fig. 2.** Estimated annual in-hospital cases of rFVIIa use for hemophilia and off-label indications. Cases signify the number of hospitalizations during which rFVIIa was used. All cases for each year are depicted. The width of each segment represents the number of cases for each category, as indicated by differential shading. Hemophilia includes hemophilia A and B, and trauma includes body and brain trauma. (*From* Logan AC, Yank V, Stafford RS. Off-label use of recombinant factor VIIa in U.S. hospitals: analysis of hospital records. Ann Int Med 2011;154:516–22; with permission.)

normalization of INR and whether patient outcomes are improved.[73] The uncertainty on whether the demonstrable effects of rFVIIa on INR correction are accompanied by adequate restoration of thrombin generation compared with PCCs is the cited reason why two guidelines[41,43] and one evidence-based review[73] have recommended against the routine use of rFVIIa for warfarin reversal in patients with ICH.[41]

The safety profile of rFVIIa in controlled trials in patients with spontaneous ICH suggests that an increased risk of thrombotic arterial events may be underreported by treating physicians.[74] Thromboembolic events associated with rFVIIa were reported to the FDA in approximately 2% of treated patients in clinical trials, but sufficient data were not available to identify the incidence in patients who received rFVIIa for warfarin reversal.[75] A careful case review of 285 trauma patients revealed that 27 (9.4%) had thromboembolic complications after administration of rFVIIa, including 3 patients who were treated for warfarin reversal.[76] Levi and colleagues[77] recently analyzed 35 randomized trials with 4468 subjects and found that 11.1% had thromboembolic events. Rates of venous thromboembolic events were similar for subjects who received rFVIIa compared with placebo (5.3% and 5.7%, respectively); arterial events, however, were significantly higher (5.5% vs 3.2%, $P<.003$) in subjects receiving rFVIIa compared with placebo, particularly for older patients and/or higher doses.

## EVOLVING CONSIDERATIONS

Emerging oral anticoagulant therapies such as antithrombin (dabigatran) and anti-Xa (rivaroxaban) inhibitors have presented special challenges; although their ease of use and benefit/safety profile compared with vitamin K antagonists[78,79] are leading to increased use of these new agents, there is uncertainty regarding effective ways to reverse anticoagulation in settings with critical bleeding such as ICH.[80] A drawback for these agents is the absence of an antidote when immediate reversal of the anticoagulant effect is needed regardless of the relative short half-life of these agents.[81] PCC has been reported to reverse the anticoagulant effect of rivaroxaban (factor Xa inhibitor) but not dabigatran (thrombin inhibitor) in humans.[82] Clinical trials for treatment of bleeding are needed. Similarly, potential roles for plasma or rFVIIa for reversal of these emerging anticoagulants remain undefined.

## SUMMARY

Institutional clinical care pathways are needed in order to successfully manage patients with refractory bleeding. Limitations to successful plasma therapy include constraints related to inventory, turnaround time, and volumes infused. For PCCs, approval status and availability of four-factor PCCs are limited, and three-factor PCCs are not approved for replacement of the vitamin K–dependent clotting factors, except for factor IX. Close collaboration among emergency medicine, critical care specialists, hematology, transfusion medicine, neurology/neurosurgery, and pharmacy services is necessary for patient blood management in critical care settings.

In the absence of clearly supportive evidence, for patient benefit, and with much data suggesting an increased risk of TAEs, critical care specialists should exercise restraint in the use of rFVIIa in off-label settings. Until better quality and more statistically significant data regarding the use of rFVIIa in different off-label scenarios become available, it is valuable for medical organizations to develop evidence-based guidelines for use of rFVIIa in off-label settings, which should be updated frequently to reflect findings from new clinical trials. Physicians need to be encouraged to adapt their clinical practices with sound clinical evidence for use of each of these hemostatic/prothrombotic products: plasma, PCCs, and rFVIIa. Finally, recently available and emerging plasma products such as fibrinogen concentrate therapy in cardiac surgery[83] and universal donor pooled plasma[84] are examples that offer opportunities to improve patient blood management using plasma and plasma products.

## REFERENCES

1. Young PP, Cotton BA, Goodnough LT. Massive transfusion protocols for patients with substantial hemorrhage. Trans Med Rev 2011;25:293–303.
2. Burtelow M, Riley E, Druzin M, et al. How we treat: management of life-threatening primary postpartum hemorrhage with a standardized massive transfusion protocol. Transfusion 2007;47:1564–72.
3. Tripodi A, Mannucci PM. The coagulopathy of chronic liver disease. N Engl J Med 2011;365:147–56.
4. Lisman T, Porte RJ. Rebalanced hemostasis in patients with liver disease: evidence and clinical consequences. Blood 2010;116:878–85.
5. Wehrli G, Taylor NE, Haines AL, et al. Instituting a thawed plasma procedure: it just makes sense and saves cents. Transfusion 2009;49:2625–30.
6. Smak Gregoor PJ, Harvey MS, Briet E, et al. Coagulation parameters of CPD fresh-frozen plasma and CPD cryoprecipitate-poor plasma after storage at 4 degrees C for 28 days. Transfusion 1993;33:735–8.
7. Epstein JS, Holmberg JA. Progress in monitoring blood safety. Transfusion 2010;50: 1408–12.
8. Hellstern P. Fresh-frozen plasma, pathogen-reduced single-donor plasma or bio-pharmaceutical plasma? Transfus Apher Sci 2008;39:69–74.
9. Narick C, Triulzi DJ, Yazer MH. Transfusion-associated circulatory overload after plasma transfusion. Transfusion 2012;52:160–5.
10. Shaz BH, Stowell SR, Hillyer CD. Transfusion-related acute lung injury: from bedside to bench and back. Blood 2011;117:1463–71.

11. Lin Y, Saw CL, Hannach B, et al. Transfusion-related acute lung injury prevention measures and their impact at Canadian Blood Services. Transfusion 2012;52:567–74.
12. Eder AF, Herron RM Jr, Strupp A, et al. Effective reduction of transfusion-related acute lung injury risk with male-predominant plasma strategy in the American Red Cross (2006–2008). Transfusion 2010;50:1732–42.
13. AABB Association Bulletin (#06-07): Transfusion-related acute lung injury. Bethesda (MD): AABB Press; 2006.
14. AABB. Standards for blood banks and transfusion services. 27th edition. Bethesda (MD): AABB Press; 2011.
15. Kleinman S, Grossman B, Kopko P. A national survey of transfusion-related acute lung injury risk reduction policies for platelets and plasma in the United States. Transfusion 2010;50:1312–21.
16. Goodnough LT, Daniels K, Wong AE, et al. How we treat: transfusion medicine support of obstetric services. Transfusion 2011;51:2540–8.
17. Murad MH, Stubbs JR, Gandhi MJ, et al. The effect of plasma transfusion on morbidity and mortality: a systematic review and meta-analysis. Transfusion 2010;50:1370–83.
18. Roback JD, Caldwell S, Carson J, et al. Evidence-based practice guidelines for plasma transfusion. Transfusion 2010;50:1227–39.
19. Segal JB, Dzik WH. Paucity of studies to support that abnormal coagulation test results predict bleeding in the setting of invasive procedures: an evidence-based review. Transfusion 2005;45:1413–25.
20. Sjoblom L, Hardemark HG, Lindgren A, et al. Management and prognostic features of intracerebral hemorrhage during anticoagulant therapy: a Swedish multicenter study. Stroke 2001;32:2567–74.
21. Goodnough LT, Shander A. How I treat warfarin-associated coagulopathy in patients with intracerebral hemorrhage. Blood 2011;117:6091–9.
22. Ewe K. Bleeding after liver biopsy does not correlate with indices of peripheral coagulation. Dig Dis Sci 1981;26:388–93.
23. Tripodi A, Caldwell SH, Hoffman M, et al. Review article: the prothrombin time test as a measure of bleeding risk and prognosis in liver disease. Aliment Pharmacol Ther 2007;26:141–8.
24. Boks AL, Brommer EJ, Schalm SW, et al. Hemostasis and fibrinolysis in severe liver failure and their relation to hemorrhage. Hepatology 1986;6:79–86.
25. Tripodi A, Primignani M, Chantarangkul V, et al. Thrombin generation in patients with cirrhosis: the role of platelets. Hepatology 2006;44:440–5.
26. Tripodi A, Primignani M, Lemma L, et al. Detection of the imbalance of procoagulant versus anticoagulant factors in cirrhosis by a simple laboratory method. Hepatology 2010;52:249–55.
27. Youssef WI, Salazar F, Dasarathy S, et al. Role of fresh frozen plasma infusion in correction of coagulopathy of chronic liver disease: a dual phase study. Am J Gastroenterol 2003;98:1391–4.
28. Sharara AI, Rockey DC. Gastroesophageal variceal hemorrhage. N Engl J Med 2001;345:669–81.
29. Holland L, Warkentin TE, Refaai M, et al. Suboptimal effect of a three-factor prothrombin complex concentrate (Profilnine-SD) in correcting supratherapeutic international normalized ratio due to warfarin overdose. Transfusion 2009;49:1171–7.
30. Pabinger I, Brenner B, Kalina U, et al. Prothrombin complex concentrate (Beriplex P/N) for emergency anticoagulation reversal: a prospective multinational clinical trial. J Thromb Haemost 2008;6:622–31.

31. Efficacy and safety study of BERIPLEX® P/N compared with plasma in patients with acute major bleeding caused by anticoagulant therapy. Available at: http://clinicaltrials. gov/ct2/show/study/NCT00708435. Accessed December 6, 2011.

32. Douketis JD. Perioperative management of patients receiving anticoagulant or anti-platelet therapy: a clinician-oriented and practical approach. Hosp Pract (Minneap) 2011;39:41–54.

33. Imberti D, Barillari G, Biasioli C, et al. Emergency reversal of anticoagulation with a three-factor prothrombin complex concentrate in patients with intracranial haemor-rhage. Blood Transfus 2011;9:148–55.

34. Lorenz R, Kienast J, Otto U, et al. Successful emergency reversal of phenprocoumon anticoagulation with prothrombin complex concentrate: a prospective clinical study. Blood Coagul Fibrinolysis 2007;18:565–70.

35. Goldstein JN, Rosand J, Schwamm LH. Warfarin reversal in anticoagulant-associated intracerebral hemorrhage. Neurocrit Care 2008;9:277–83.

36. Wiedermann CJ, Stockner I. Warfarin-induced bleeding complications - clinical pre-sentation and therapeutic options. Thromb Res 2008;122(Suppl 2):S13–8.

37. Makris M, van Veen JJ, Maclean R. Warfarin anticoagulation reversal: management of the asymptomatic and bleeding patient. J Thromb Thrombolysis 2010;29:171–81.

38. Bershad EM, Suarez JI. Prothrombin complex concentrates for oral anticoagulant therapy-related intracranial hemorrhage: a review of the literature. Neurocrit Care 2010;12:403–13.

39. Baker RI, Coughlin PB, Gallus AS, et al. Warfarin reversal: consensus guidelines, on behalf of the Australasian Society of Thrombosis and Haemostasis. Med J Aust 2004;181:492–7.

40. Steiner T, Kaste M, Forsting M, et al. Recommendations for the management of intracranial haemorrhage - part I: spontaneous intracerebral haemorrhage. The Eu-ropean Stroke Initiative Writing Committee and the Writing Committee for the EUSI Executive Committee. Cerebrovasc Dis 2006;22:294–316.

41. Morgenstern LB, Hemphill JC 3rd, Anderson C, et al. Guidelines for the management of spontaneous intracerebral hemorrhage: a guideline for healthcare professionals from the American Heart Association/American Stroke Association. Stroke 2010;41: 2108–29.

42. Pernod G, Godier A, Gozalo C, et al. French clinical practice guidelines on the management of patients on vitamin K antagonists in at-risk situations (overdose, risk of bleeding, and active bleeding). Thromb Res 2010;126:e167–74.

43. Keeling D, Baglin T, Tait C, et al. Guidelines on oral anticoagulation with warfarin-fourth edition. Br J Haematol 2011;154:311–24.

44. Ageno W, Gallus AS, Wittkowsky A, et al. Oral anticoagulant therapy: Antithrombotic Therapy and Prevention of Thrombosis, 9th ed: American College of Chest Physicians Evidence-Based Clinical Practice Guidelines. Chest 2012;141:e44S–88S.

45. Beshay JE, Morgan H, Madden C, et al. Emergency reversal of anticoagulation and antiplatelet therapies in neurosurgical patients. J Neurosurg 2010;112:307–18.

46. Marietta M, Pedrazzi P, Luppi M. Three- or four-factor prothrombin complex concen-trate for emergency anticoagulation reversal: what are we really looking for? Blood Transfus 2011;9:469.

47. Hellstern P. Production and composition of prothrombin complex concentrates: correlation between composition and therapeutic efficiency. Thromb Res 1999;95: S7–12.

48. Warkentin TE, Crowther MA. Reversing anticoagulants both old and new. Can J Anaesth 2002;49:S11–25.

49. FEIBA NF (anti-inhibitor coagulant complex). 2010. Available at: http://www.fda.gov/ BiologicsBloodVaccines/BloodBloodProducts/ApprovedProducts/Licensed ProductsBLAs/FractionatedPlasmaProducts/ucm221726.htm. Accessed December 7, 2011.

50. Wojcik C, Schymik ML, Cure EG. Activated prothrombin complex concentrate factor VIII inhibitor bypassing activity (FEIBA) for the reversal of warfarin-induced coagulopathy. Int J Emerg Med 2009;2:217–25.

51. Bobbitt L, Merriman E, Raynes J, et al. PROTHROMBINEX(®)-VF (PTX-VF) usage for reversal of coagulopathy: prospective evaluation of thrombogenic risk. Thromb Res 2011;128:577–82.

52. Grottke O, Braunschweig T, Spronk HM, et al. Increasing concentrations of prothrombin complex concentrate induce disseminated intravascular coagulation in a pig model of coagulopathy with blunt liver injury. Blood 2011;118:1943–51.

53. Lusher JM. Thrombogenicity associated with factor IX complex concentrates. Semin Hematol 1991;28:3–5.

54. Kohler M. Thrombogenicity of prothrombin complex concentrates. Thromb Res 1999;95:S13–7.

55. Bui JD, Despotis GD, Trulock EP, et al. Fatal thrombosis after administration of activated prothrombin complex concentrates in a patient supported by extracorporeal membrane oxygenation who had received activated recombinant factor VII. J Thorac Cardiovasc Surg 2002;124:852–4.

56. Warren O, Simon B. Massive, fatal, intracardiac thrombosis associated with prothrombin complex concentrate. Ann Emerg Med 2009;53:758–61.

57. Riess HB, Meier-Hellmann A, Motsch J, et al. Prothrombin complex concentrate (Octaplex) in patients requiring immediate reversal of oral anticoagulation. Thromb Res 2007;121:9–16.

58. Pabinger I, Tiede A, Kalina U, et al. Impact of infusion speed on the safety and effectiveness of prothrombin complex concentrate: a prospective clinical trial of emergency anticoagulation reversal. Ann Hematol 2010;89:309–16.

59. Franchini M, Lippi G. Prothrombin complex concentrates: an update. Blood Transfus 2010;8:149–54.

60. Khorsand N, Veeger NJ, Muller M, et al. Fixed versus variable dose of prothrombin complex concentrate for counteracting vitamin K antagonist therapy. Transfus Med 2011;21:116–23.

61. Ratnoff OD. Some complications of the therapy of classic hemophilia. J Lab Clin Med 1984;103:653–9.

62. Heger A, Svae TE, Neisser-Svae A, et al. Biochemical quality of the pharmaceutically licensed plasma OctaplasLG after implementation of a novel prion protein (PrPSc) removal technology and reduction of the solvent/detergent (S/D) process time. Vox Sang 2009;97:219–25.

63. Custer B, Agapova M, Martinez RH. The cost-effectiveness of pathogen reduction technology as assessed using a multiple risk reduction model. Transfusion 2010;50: 2461–73.

64. Toner RW, Pizzi L, Leas B, et al. Costs to hospitals of acquiring and processing blood in the US: a survey of hospital-based blood banks and transfusion services. Appl Health Econ Health Policy 2011;9:29–37.

65. Poon MC. Use of recombinant factor VIIa in hereditary bleeding disorders. Curr Opin Hematol 2001;8:312–8.

66. Logan AC, Yank V, Stafford RS. Off-Label use of recombinant factor VIIa in U.S. hospitals: analysis of hospital records. Ann Intern Med 2011;154:516–22.

67. Goodnough LT, Lublin DM, Zhang L, et al. Transfusion medicine service policies for recombinant factor VIIa administration. Transfusion 2004;44:1325–31.
68. Yank V, Tuohy CV, Logan AC, et al. Systematic review: benefits and harms of in-hospital use of recombinant factor VIIa for off-label indications. Ann Intern Med 2011;154:529–40.
69. Freeman WD, Brott TG, Barrett KM, et al. Recombinant factor VIIa for rapid reversal of warfarin anticoagulation in acute intracranial hemorrhage. Mayo Clin Proc 2004;79: 1495–500.
70. Ilyas C, Beyer GM, Dutton RP, et al. Recombinant factor VIIa for warfarin-associated intracranial bleeding. J Clin Anesth 2008;20:276–9.
71. Robinson MT, Rabinstein AA, Meschia JF, et al. Safety of recombinant activated factor VII in patients with warfarin-associated hemorrhages of the central nervous system. Stroke 2010;41:1459–63.
72. Deveras RA, Kessler CM. Reversal of warfarin-induced excessive anticoagulation with recombinant human factor VIIa concentrate. Ann Intern Med 2002;137:884–8.
73. Rosovsky RP, Crowther MA. What is the evidence for the off-label use of recombinant factor VIIa (rFVIIa) in the acute reversal of warfarin? ASH evidence-based review 2008. Hematology Am Soc Hematol Educ Program 2008:36–8.
74. Logan AC, Goodnough LT. Recombinant factor VIIa: an assessment of evidence regarding its efficacy and safety in the off-label setting. Hematology Am Soc Hematol Educ Program 2010;2010:153–9.
75. O'Connell KA, Wood JJ, Wise RP, et al. Thromboembolic adverse events after use of recombinant human coagulation factor VIIa. JAMA 2006;295:293–8.
76. Thomas GO, Dutton RP, Hemlock B, et al. Thromboembolic complications associated with factor VIIa administration. J Trauma 2007;62:564–9.
77. Levi M, Levy JH, Andersen HF, et al. Safety of recombinant activated factor VII in randomized clinical trials. N Engl J Med 2010;363:1791–800.
78. Bauersachs R, Berkowitz SD, Brenner B, et al. Oral rivaroxaban for symptomatic venous thromboembolism. N Engl J Med 2010;363:2499–510.
79. Schulman S, Kearon C, Kakkar AK, et al. Dabigatran versus warfarin in the treatment of acute venous thromboembolism. N Engl J Med 2009;361:2342–52.
80. van Ryn J, Stangier J, Haertter S, et al. Dabigatran etexilate–a novel, reversible, oral direct thrombin inhibitor: interpretation of coagulation assays and reversal of anticoagulant activity. Thromb Haemost 2010;103:1116–27.
81. Crowther MA, Warkentin TE. Managing bleeding in anticoagulated patients with a focus on novel therapeutic agents. J Thromb Haemost 2009;7(Suppl 1):107–10.
82. Eerenberg ES, Kamphuisen PW, Sijpkens MK, et al. Reversal of rivaroxaban and dabigatran by prothrombin complex concentrate: a randomized, placebo-controlled, crossover study in healthy subjects. Circulation 2011;124:1573–9.
83. Karlsson M, Ternstrom L, Hyllner M, et al. Prophylactic fibrinogen infusion reduces bleeding after coronary artery bypass surgery. A prospective randomised pilot study. Thromb Haemost 2009;102:137–44.
84. Heger A, Romisch J, Svae TE. A biochemical comparison of a pharmaceutically licensed coagulation active plasma (Octaplas) with a universally applicable development product (Uniplas) and single-donor FFPs subjected to methylene-blue dye and white-light treatment. Transfus Apher Sci 2006;35:223–33.

# Newer Anticoagulants in Critically Ill Patients

Anita Rajasekhar, MD[a], Rebecca Beyth, MD, MSc[a],
Mark A. Crowther, MD, MSc, FRCPC[b],*

## KEYWORDS

- Anticoagulants • Critical care • Thrombosis • Pharmacology

## KEY POINTS

- While critically ill patients are at increased risk for development of thrombosis, they are particularly susceptible to bleeding complications from anticoagulants.
- Rigorous clinical trials of newer anticoagulants in critically ill patients are lacking.
- Clinicians should be aware of the indications, pharmacology, methods for monitoring anticoagulant activity, and recommendations for management of bleeding and perioperative use of these newer anticoagulants.

## INTRODUCTION

Anticoagulants are unique compared with most pharmacologic agents because even small deviations from therapeutic levels place patients at risk for life-threatening complications. Whereas critically ill patients are particularly susceptible to thrombosis, they also have higher risks of bleeding than the general medical or surgical patients. Although the choices for anticoagulant therapy are expanding with the development of new parenteral and oral agents, rigorous clinical trials of their use in the intensive care unit (ICU) population are lacking. The authors discuss the use of newer anticoagulants in the ICU population including pharmacology, evidence from clinical trials leading to approved indications, management of bleeding, and perioperative use of the newer anticoagulants.

## NEWER ANTICOAGULANTS: PHARMACOLOGY AND EVIDENCE FROM CLINICAL TRIALS

### Low-Molecular-Weight Heparins

Low-molecular-weight heparins (LMWHs) exert their anticoagulant effects by binding to antithrombin, thereby enhancing its capacity to inhibit thrombin and factor Xa.[1]

[a] Department of Medicine, University of Florida, College of Medicine, Health Science Center, PO Box 00278, Gainesville, FL 32610-0278, USA; [b] Department of Medicine, McMaster University, St Joseph's Hospital, Room H303, 50 Charlton Avenue East, Hamilton, Ontario L8N 4A6, Canada
* Corresponding author.
E-mail address: crowthrm@mcmaster.ca

Crit Care Clin 28 (2012) 427–451
http://dx.doi.org/10.1016/j.ccc.2012.04.005
0749-0704/12/$ – see front matter © 2012 Published by Elsevier Inc.

criticalcare.theclinics.com

This inhibition of factor Xa is mediated by a unique pentasaccharide sequence found on about one-fifth of LMWH chains. The interaction of heparin with thrombin also requires the pentasaccharide sequence in concert with a heparin molecule of sufficient length to simultaneously bind to both antithrombin and thrombin. The mean molecular weight of LMWH is 5000 Da. Therefore, in contrast to the larger unfractionated heparin (UFH) molecule (mean mass of 15,000 Da), most of the LMWH chains are insufficient in length to bridge antithrombin to thrombin. Thus, LMWH catalyzes the inhibition of factor Xa to a greater extent than thrombin.[1]

LMWH has a more predictable anticoagulant effect than heparin because of less plasma protein binding. The half-life of LMWH ranges from 2 to 5 hours depending on the specific LMWH used. Bioavailability after subcutaneous (SQ) injection is approximately 90%, and peak concentrations are reached at 1 to 5 hours. LMWH does not reliably alter the activated partial thromboplastin time (aPTT) or prothrombin time (PT) at therapeutic concentrations. Because the clearance of LMWHs is primarily through the kidney, bioaccumulation of some LMWHs may occur in patients with creatinine clearance (CrCl) less than 30 mL/min. Protamine sulfate only partially reverses the anticoagulant effect of LMWH. Because longer chains bind protamine with higher affinity, protamine reverses all of the anti-IIa (antithrombin) activity of LMWH but only 60% of LMWH's anti-Xa activity.[1] The dose of protamine varies based on LMWH subtype (1 mg protamine per 100 mg enoxaparin or 1 mg protamine per 100 U of dalteparin or tinzaparin)[1,2] (**Table 1**).

Currently available LMWHs include enoxaparin, dalteparin, and tinzaparin. Traditionally LMWHs have several advantages over UFH such as better bioavailability and more predictable dose response. Consequently, LMWH can be given as a once- or twice-daily dose without routine monitoring. This regimen allows for more convenient administration, such as outpatient management of venous thromboembolism (VTE). Other safety advantages over UFH include a decreased incidence of heparin-induced thrombocytopenia (HIT) due to less binding to platelet factor 4. Furthermore, the risk of osteoporosis with long-term LMWH use is thought to be less than UFH because of reduced binding to osteoblasts.[1,3] These properties make LMWH an attractive alternative to UFH anticoagulation in the general population.

In contrast, the use of LMWHs in the ICU setting may be more problematic, because these patients often have comorbidities (obesity, renal insufficiency/failure, anasarca, or hypotension requiring inotrope therapy), which can lead to unpredictable dose effects. If levels fall outside the usual therapeutic range as a result of these abnormalities, patients may be placed at risk for underdosing (causing avoidable thrombosis) or overdosing (causing avoidable bleeding). Because of their long half-lives compared with UFH, especially in patients with renal impairment, LMWH to produce therapeutic anticoagulation (in contrast to prophylactic anticoagulation) is rarely used in ICU patients. However, in the PROTECT study, which compared 5000 units of dalteparin once daily to UFH 5000 units twice daily for VTE prophylaxis in critically ill patients, there was no difference in the rates of major bleeding (5.5% vs 5.6 %, respectively) despite the inclusion of patients with a range of renal insufficiency, including patients with end-stage renal disease requiring hemodialysis.[4] Similarly, the incidence of major bleeding was investigated in the IRIS study that included renally impaired elderly patients aged 70 years or older with acute symptomatic lower extremity deep vein thrombosis (DVT) requiring therapeutic dose anticoagulation. Patients were randomized to initial treatment with either tinzaparin or UFH. Although the study was stopped early because of a difference in mortality favoring the UFH group, the rates of major bleeding at 90 days were no different between the two groups (4.5% vs 3.7%, respectively; $P = .68$).[5] In contrast, an earlier metaanalysis of

**Table 1**
Pharmacologic properties of heparin and its derivatives

| Properties | Unfractionated Heparin | LMWH | Specific Anti-Xa Inhibitor |
|---|---|---|---|
| Types | | Enoxaparin, dalteparin, tinzaparin | Fondaparinux |
| Molecular weight | 15,000 Da | 5000 Da | 1500 Da |
| Target | FIIa and FXa | FXa > FIIa | FXa only |
| Bioavailability | 30% | 90% | 100% |
| Time to peak concentration | IV; immediate SQ: 20–60 min | ~1.5 h | ~2 h |
| Half-life | ~1.5 h | ~2.5 h | ~17–21 h |
| Elimination | Reticuloendothelial system | Renal | Renal |
| Reversible | Complete with protamine | Partially with protamine | No |
| Laboratory monitoring | aPTT, anti-Xa heparin levels | Not required, can measure anti-Xa LMWH levels | Not required, can measure anti-Xa fondaparinux levels |
| Potential for HIT | <5% | <1% | No |

*Abbreviations:* FIIa, factor IIa; FXa, factor Xa; HIT, heparin-induced thrombocytopenia; IV, intravenous.

12 studies involving approximately 5000 patients revealed that therapeutic enoxaparin dosing was associated with increase in major bleeding in patients with a CrCl of 30 mL/min or less compared with UFH (8.3% vs 2.4%, respectively; 95% confidence interval [CI], 1.78–8.45).[6]

These observations suggest that when used at prophylactic doses, dalteparin and tinzaparin are unlikely to bioaccumulate, and they can be safely used at usual doses. However, enoxaparin may bioaccumulate and should be used at a reduced dose (30 mg SQ once daily) for VTE prophylaxis. When used at therapeutic doses, however, there is little or no evidence for guiding dosing regimens in critically ill patients. Consequently, when these agents are used in critically ill patients, particularly those with renal failure, the authors suggest clinicians consider monitoring the anticoagulant effect with anti-Xa heparin levels 4 hours after the third dose (when steady state has been achieved) to assess for potential increased drug accumulation. Furthermore, repeat anti-Xa levels are warranted after any dose adjustments or changes in renal function. The target therapeutic range (in anti-Xa units) is .5 to 1.0 U/mL for patients on twice-daily LMWH and 1.0 to 2.0 U/mL for patients on once-daily LMWH. Although these agents are as effective as UFH for the treatment and prevention of acute VTE, clinical trials have generally excluded ICU patients. Therefore, the efficacy and safety of LMWHs in the treatment of acute VTE in critically ill patients remains unclear.

Danaparoid is a heparinoid that is used predominately in the care of patients with suspected heparin-induced thrombocytopenia. It is no longer available in the United States and will not be discussed further here.

### Indirect Anti-Xa Inhibitors

Fondaparinux is a synthetic analog of the antithrombin-binding pentasaccharide sequence found in UFH and LMWH. As a synthetic drug, fondaparinux may be safer than UFH and LMWH, which are derived from animal byproducts. Fondaparinux has a higher affinity for antithrombin compared with UFH or LMWH. Its chain length is too short to bridge antithrombin to thrombin and therefore, unlike UFH and LMWH, fondaparinux is a highly specific inhibitor of factor Xa. Fondaparinux is almost 100% bioavailable 2 hours after SQ injection. As the lowest molecular weight heparin derivative, fondaparinux does not bind to other plasma proteins, platelets, or the endothelium, thereby creating even more of a predictable dose-response effect than LMWH. Its lack of binding to proteins suggests it should not cause heparin-induced thrombocytopenia, which is caused by the binding of heparin to a platelet-derived protein, known as platelet factor 4. However, there have been rare case reports implicating this agent in the development of HIT. The half-life of fondaparinux is approximately 18 hours allowing for once-daily dosing. It is renally cleared and therefore is contraindicated in patients with a CrCl less than 30 mL/min. Fondaparinux does not alter the aPTT or PT at therapeutic concentrations. Because of the short chain length of fondaparinux, protamine cannot be used for its reversal.[7–9]

Fondaparinux is currently approved for (1) thromboprophylaxis following hip and knee arthroplasty and hip fracture surgery and (2) the initial treatment of VTE.[10] However, studies that led to these US Food and Drug Administration (FDA)-approved indications excluded critically ill patients and patients with important degrees of organ dysfunction. Because of its long half-life, inability to reverse the anticoagulant effects, and the propensity of ICU patients to have renal insufficiency and higher bleeding risk, fondaparinux is rarely used in this population for the treatment or prevention of VTE (see **Table 1**). Fondaparinux is highly effective for the treatment of acute coronary syndromes (ACS).[11] However, even in the low doses used for ACS treatment, there is a risk of bioaccumulation suggesting that extreme care should be used if fondaparinux is being considered in critically ill patients with ACS. UFH may be a safer alternative in this setting.

### Parenteral Direct Thrombin Inhibitors

Parenteral direct thrombin inhibitors (DTIs) such as lepirudin, bivalirudin, and arga-troban, are based on antithrombin-*independent* inhibition of thrombin. DTIs bind directly to free and fibrin-bound thrombin and inhibit the multiple actions of thrombin including activation of protein C, proinflammatory cytokines, and thrombin-activatable fibrinolysis inhibitor. These drugs interfere with thrombin-dependent clot-based tests. Specifically, each DTI prolongs the aPTT, PT, and international normalized ratio (INR) to varying degrees. These clot-based tests remain prolonged in mixing studies as seen with other clotting factor inhibitors. The thrombin time/thrombin clotting time (TT/TCT) is too sensitive at therapeutic concentrations of DTI to use for monitoring. Therefore, DTIs are typically monitored with the aPTT. However, clinicians must consider confounding factors that prolong the baseline aPTT (factor deficiencies, lupus anticoagulant, severe vitamin K deficiency), especially in the ICU population. DTIs have a more predictable anticoagulant effect compared with heparins because they do not bind plasma proteins in circulation, have antiplatelet effects, or induce an immune-mediated thrombocytopenia.[12] No reversal agent currently exists for these DTIs. Currently four parenteral DTIs are approved for use in the United States: argatroban, lepirudin, desirudin, and bivalirudin. The pharmacologic and clinical properties of each DTI are summarized in **Table 2**.

Argatroban is the primary DTI used in the ICU setting. Argatroban is approved for the prophylaxis or treatment of thrombosis complicating HIT and in patients with/at risk for HIT undergoing percutaneous coronary intervention (PCI).[10] It is a reversible synthetic thrombin inhibitor derived from L-arginine. It has a short half-life (45 minutes), making it an attractive anticoagulant in patients with high risk of bleeding. Because of hepatic metabolism, dose adjustments are required for hepatic impairment but not renal insufficiency. The starting dose in patients without liver dysfunction is 2 $\mu$g/kg/min and does not require a bolus injection. With moderate liver dysfunction (Child-Pugh score 7–11) the starting dose should be reduced to .5 $\mu$g/kg/min.[13,14] Dose adjustments are made based on aPTT with a goal aPTT of 1.5 to 3 times normal range. The aPTT should be monitored 2 hours after initiation of therapy or with dose adjustments. If the aPTT is elevated (>100 seconds) the infusion should be temporarily stopped until the aPTT returns to goal range. Argatroban can then be restarted at 50% of the previous dose. Argatroban is contraindicated in patients with hepatic insufficiency. In critically ill patients with multiorgan failure, an initial dose reduction to .2 $\mu$g/kg/min is recommended.[15] Argatroban can cause pronounced prolongation of the PT/INR compared with the other parenteral DTIs. In the setting of HIT this prolongation of INR can result in difficulties when transitioning to warfarin therapy, with the risk of stopping argatroban too early. The following is recommended when transitioning from argatroban to warfarin therapy and is summarized in **Fig. 1**:

1. First, concomitant vitamin K deficiency should be treated simultaneously to prevent synergistic elevation in the INR.
2. Argatroban should be administered parallel to warfarin for at least 5 days and until the INR exceeds 4.
3. Argatroban can then be stopped and the INR rechecked 4 to 6 hours later.
4. If the INR remains at therapeutic range, warfarin can then be continued at current dose.

**Table 2**
Pharmacologic properties of the parenteral direct thrombin inhibitors

| Properties | Argatroban | Lepirudin | Desirudin | Bivalirudin |
|---|---|---|---|---|
| Half-life | ~45 min | ~80 min | ~120 min | ~25 min |
| Elimination | Hepatic | Renal | Renal | Enzymatic, 20% renal |
| Antidote | No | No | No | No |
| Laboratory monitoring | aPTT, ACT | aPTT, ACT | Not required, can monitor aPTT | aPTT, ACT |
| Prolongation of INR | Significant | Minor | Minor | Minor |
| Dose reductions | Moderate hepatic impairment: .5 µg/kg/min in HIT<br>Severe HF: CI | CrCl 15–60 mL/min: 15%–50% DR<br>CrCl <15 mL/min: CI | CrCl <31–60 mL/min: DR unnecessary | CrCl 15–60 mL/min: 15%–50% DR<br>CrCl <15 mL/min: CI |
| FDA indications | (1) Prophylaxis or treatment of thrombosis complicating HIT<br>(2) HIT with or without thrombosis undergoing PCI | (1) Prophylaxis or treatment of thrombosis complicating HIT | (1) DVT prevention after THR | (1) Unstable angina undergoing PTCA<br>(2) PCI with provisional use of GPI<br>(3) HIT with or without thrombosis undergoing PCI |

*Abbreviations:* ACT, activated clotting time; CI, contraindicated; DR, dose reduction; GPI, glycoprotein inhibitor; HF, heart failure; PCI, percutaneous coronary interventions; PTCA, percutaneous transluminal coronary angioplasty; THR, total hip replacement.

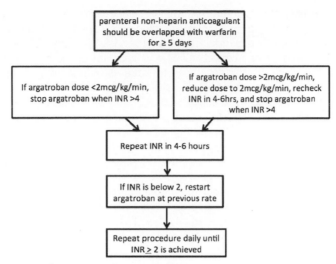

**Fig. 1.** Transitioning from argatroban to warfarin.

5. If the INR is below 2.0, argatroban should then be reinitiated and the dose of warfarin increased with the INR rechecked the following day.[16]

Lepirudin is a recombinant derivative of hirudin that is FDA-approved for the prophylaxis or treatment of thrombosis complicating HIT.[10] It is a bivalent inhibitor, acting at both the exosite 1 domain and active site of thrombin. Dosing is based on body weight and adjustments made based on aPTT, although activated clotting time (ACT) is used for monitoring in the setting of cardiopulmonary bypass. Lepirudin has several limitations that may preclude its use in the ICU: predominant renal clearance, narrow therapeutic window, increased bleeding events, and potential formation of antihirudin antibodies following treatment of HIT, which may further delay renal clearance.[16–19] Rarely, anaphylaxis has been reported in patients who develop antibodies and are reexposed to hirudin.[19] After April 2012, the manufacturer (Celgene) has discontinued lepirudin from the market, although not for safety concerns.[20]

Desirudin is also a recombinant derivative of the naturally occurring hirudin. It is the only fixed-dose (15 mg SQ twice daily) subcutaneously administered DTI available and does not require laboratory monitoring unless there is an increased risk of bleeding. Desirudin has a rapid onset of action (ie, within 30 minutes) and reaches peak plasma concentrations within1 to 3 hours after SQ administration. Its half-life is approximately 2 hours. Desirudin's anticoagulant activity can be measured by aPTT and TT/TCT. Because of predominant excretion by the kidneys (80%–90%), dose reductions and monitoring with aPTT are recommended for renal impairment (CrCl < 30 mL/min).[18,21] Desirudin is approved for thromboprophylaxis against VTE after elective total hip replacement.[10,22] Two studies involving 1938 patients undergoing elective hip replacement found that desirudin was superior in comparison with UFH 5000 units SQ three times daily or enoxaparin 40 mg SQ daily for prevention of postoperative DVT.[23,24] The safety profile of desirudin was similar to UFH and enoxaparin. Desirudin has also been studied in acute myocardial infarction, in unstable angina, and in hemodialysis.[25–28] In the TIMI 9B trial, UFH and desirudin as an adjunct to thrombolytics was equally effective in preventing death, recurrent nonfatal myocardial infarction, and development of severe congestive heart failure or cardiogenic shock.[25] Similar rates of major bleeding were observed in each group. In the GUSTO IIb trial, desirudin reduced the risk of early (24-hour) nonfatal myocardial infarction compared with UFH and was not associated with increased bleeding risk.[26] Finally, in another study of patients with chronic renal failure on maintenance dialysis, desirudin was equally effective as UFH as an anticoagulant during dialysis.[28] Desirudin's efficacy, safety, and cost-effectiveness are being investigated in the PREVENT-HIT study as an alternative to argatroban in the treatment of HIT with or without thrombosis.[29]

Bivalirudin is a synthetically engineered analog of hirudin that reversibly inhibits exosite 1 domain and the active site of thrombin. Bivalirudin demonstrates several advantageous properties including reversible binding to thrombin and thus less bleeding risk,[30] enzymatic metabolism, immediate onset of action (5 minutes), short half-life (25 minutes), monitoring with widely available testing (ACT or aPTT), minimal effect on the INR, and low immunogenicity. Bivalirudin is predominantly metabolized by proteolysis. Dose adjustments are required for moderate renal insufficiency because 20% is excreted unchanged by the kidneys. Antibodies to bivalirudin are rarely detected. Bivalirudin is FDA-approved for (1) unstable angina undergoing percutaneous transluminal coronary angioplasty, (2) PCI with provisional use of glycoprotein IIb/IIIa inhibitor, and (3) as an alternative to UFH in suspected HIT patients with or without thrombosis undergoing PCI.[10]

Whereas these parenteral agents serve as potential alternatives to conventional anticoagulants (UFH, LMWH, fondaparinux), their safety and efficacy in comparison with UFH and LMWHs in the ICU population have yet to be defined. Currently, the primary clinical use of these agents in the critically ill is in the realm of suspected or proven HIT, with argatroban being the preferred DTI because of lack of renal clearance. The rapid onset of anticoagulation in combination with the lack of cross-reaction with HIT antibodies makes DTI the primary choice for alternative aggressive anticoagulation in the setting of HIT. For the treatment of HIT with or without thrombosis, the 2012 American College of Chest Physicians (ACCP) guidelines recommend the use of lepirudin, argatroban, or bivalirudin (for urgent cardiac surgery).[31]

### New Oral Anticoagulants

None of the new oral anticoagulants have been studied in the ICU population. Patients with renal and hepatic failure were systematically excluded from clinical trials that have led to approval of these agents. Nonetheless, intensivists may be faced with patients who are taking these drugs and are admitted to the ICU, or may be forced to use these agents in the treatment of selected patients. These drugs may lead to ICU admission, for example in a patient admitted with bleeding complications. Therefore, clinicians should be aware of the indications, pharmacology, methods for monitoring anticoagulant activity, and recommendations for management of bleeding with these new oral anticoagulants.

Dabigatran is a novel competitive direct thrombin inhibitor. The bioavailability of its oral prodrug is approximately 3% to 7%, with peak plasma concentrations recorded approximately 1.5 hours following oral ingestion. The half-life of dabigatran with normal renal function is 12 to 14 hours, allowing for once- or twice-daily dosing. Approximately 80% of the drug is renally cleared. Dose reductions are recommended with a CrCl of 15 to 30 mL/min. Dabigatran is contraindicated in patients with severe renal insufficiency (CrCl <15 mL/min).[32,33] Dabigatran and its prodrug are not affected by cytochrome P450 drug metabolizing enzymes. However, potential drug interactions can occur with many drugs that ICU patients are exposed to such as the

P-glycoprotein inhibitors amiodarone, verapamil, and quinidine, all of which may increase dabigatran levels.

The predictable pharmacologic properties and lower potential for drug interactions compared with warfarin allow for fixed dosing of dabigatran without the need for routine laboratory monitoring.[34–37] However, in specific clinical scenarios such as management of life-threatening hemorrhage, a readily available and simple laboratory test to assess the anticoagulant effect of dabigatran would be useful. At therapeutic doses, dabigatran prolongs the aPTT, TT/TCT, and ecarin clotting time (ECT).[37] Because of the practical limitations of obtaining ECT and TT/TCT in real time, the aPTT, although relatively insensitive, may be the more useful measure of dabigatran activity. Dabigatran has little effect on the PT at clinically relevant plasma concentrations.[37] Whereas the TT/TCT and aPTT are the most effective and widely available coagulation assays to determine presence of a dabigatran effect, the therapeutic range of these tests is not well-defined, and the tests are best used to determine the presence or absence of the drug. Therefore, clinicians should not routinely use these laboratory assays to monitor and adjust dabigatran doses or assess the degree of bleeding risk for surgical procedures. In an emergency, a normal thrombin time rules out the presence of significant amounts of dabigatran. A high-normal aPTT may be seen in patients with detectable dabigatran levels. Commercial dabigatran testing kits are available; the kits quantify dabigatran levels but are not widely available and are not currently licensed in the United States.

Dabigatran is FDA-approved for the prevention of stroke and systemic embolism in nonvalvular atrial fibrillation.[10] In the RELY study, two twice-daily doses of dabigatran, 110 mg and 150 mg, were compared with dose-adjusted warfarin in over 18,000 patients with nonvalvular atrial fibrillation. Both doses of dabigatran were shown to be noninferior to warfarin for prevention of stroke or systemic embolism. However, dabigatran 150 mg twice daily was found to be superior to warfarin for stroke prevention (1.11% per year vs 1.71% per year; $P<.001$; relative risk [RR]: .65; 95% CI: .52–.81). There was no difference in annual major bleeding rates on dabigatran compared with warfarin (3.32% per year vs 3.57% per year; $P = .32$; RR: .93; CI: .81–1.07).[38] An unexplained increase in myocardial infarction was noted in dabigatran compared with warfarin (annual risk .74% vs .53%, respectively; $P = .048$); this increase is possibly due to dabigatran not sharing warfarin's well-known protective effect against myocardial infarction.

Dabigatran has been studied in the setting of VTE prophylaxis after total knee arthroplasty[39] and total hip arthroplasty.[40] Dabigatran was found to be noninferior to enoxaparin 40 mg daily but failed to achieve noninferiority when compared with enoxaparin 30 mg twice daily. Bleeding rates were similar to enoxaparin. Based on these data, dabigatran was approved in Europe and Canada for VTE prevention after total knee arthroplasty and total hip arthroplasty.

In the RECOVER trial, patients with acute symptomatic proximal DVT or pulmonary embolism (PE) were randomized to dabigatran 150 mg twice daily or warfarin, after initial parenteral heparin. After 6 months, dabigatran was noninferior to warfarin for recurrent VTE (hazard ratio [HR] .82; 95% CI .45–1.48). Bleeding rates were also similar between the two groups, although dyspepsia was significantly higher in the dabigatran group. Because dabigatran was started only after initial parenteral therapy, as yet no evidence exists to support the initial treatment of VTE with dabigatran monotherapy.[41]

Rivaroxaban is a reversible direct factor Xa inhibitor with greater than 80% bioavailability. Peak plasma concentrations occur approximately 3 hours after oral ingestion. The half-life is 4 to 9 hours (up to 13 hours in elderly patients).

Rivaroxaban is 60% cleared by the kidneys. Whereas no specific dose reductions are given for renal insufficiency, rivaroxaban is contraindicated with CrCl less than 30 mL/min. P-glycoprotein and strong CYP3A4 inhibitors increase drug levels of rivaroxaban. Rivaroxaban is generally administered once daily. Although laboratory monitoring is not routinely required, special situations may call for measurement of anticoagulant effect. Rivaroxaban causes prolongation of both the PT and aPTT but exhibits greater sensitivity for PT. However, PT prolongation is not specific. Anti–factor Xa assays would be ideal for determining plasma rivaroxaban concentrations— commercial kits are available and levels are available in some reference coagulation laboratories. A black box warning exists for patients with neuraxial anesthesia or undergoing spinal puncture because epidural and spinal hematomas resulting in long-term or permanent paralysis have occurred.[10]

Rivaroxaban is FDA-approved for (1) prophylaxis against VTE in patients undergoing knee or hip replacement surgery and (2) to reduce the risk of stroke and systemic embolism in patients with nonvalvular atrial fibrillation.[10] Rivaroxaban was investigated in four large phase III trials for prevention of VTE after total hip and knee arthroplasty (RECORD 1-4).[42–45] In all four trials, rivaroxaban 10 mg by mouth daily was found to be superior to enoxaparin for a composite of total VTE and all-cause mortality. There were no significant differences in the rates of major bleeding or hepatic enzyme elevations between the two treatments. In the ROCKET study, approximately 14,000 patients with nonvalvular atrial fibrillation were randomly assigned to rivaroxaban 20 mg by mouth daily or dose-adjusted warfarin. Notably, patients with CrCl 30 to 50 mL/min were included in the trial with a dose reduction to 15 mg by mouth daily. Rivaroxaban was noninferior to warfarin for the prevention of stroke or systemic embolism (HR, .88; 95% CI, .74–1.03; $P<.001$ for noninferiority). There was no significant between-group difference in the risk of major bleeding, although intracranial (.5% vs .7%, $P = .02$) and fatal bleeding (.2% vs .5%, $P = .003$) occurred less frequently in the rivaroxaban group.[46] Similar to dabigatran, this new oral anticoagulant is dependent on renal function for clearance, has no effective antidote, and has not been studied rigorously in critically ill patients. Therefore its use in the intensive care unit cannot be recommended at this time.

Apixaban is a direct inhibitor of factor Xa that also has a high bioavailability (65%) after oral ingestion. Peak plasma concentrations are achieved 1 to 3 hours after intake, and the half-life is approximately 8 to 15 hours in young adults. Apixaban has little potential for drug interactions because it is metabolized through CYP-independent mechanisms.[47,48] Unlike rivaroxaban and dabigatran, apixaban is excreted primarily through nonrenal and nonhepatic mechanisms.[49] This property may lead to an advantage over dabigatran and rivaroxaban with a potential use in patients with renal or hepatic impairment. Apixaban causes dose-dependent prolongation of aPTT and PT. In situations in which monitoring is required, measuring anti–factor Xa levels would be most useful.[50]

Apixaban is currently approved by the European Commission for the prevention of VTE in patients who have undergone elective hip or knee replacement surgery. Apixaban was compared with different doses of enoxaparin in three large randomized controlled trials (ADVANCE 1–3). Taken together, the results of these three trials suggest that apixaban offers a favorable efficacy for VTE prophylaxis and similar safety profile compared with enoxaparin in patients undergoing elective hip or knee arthroplasty.[51–53] As with the other new oral anticoagulants, no evidence is available for the use of apixaban in ICU patients. Apixaban is less dependent on renal clearance than the other novel agents, making it potentially attractive in patients with renal insufficiency. However, given a lack of experience, its relatively long half-life, and the lack of an antidote for its anticoagulant effect, its use in the ICU cannot be recommended at this time.

Whereas no clinical data exist on the use of these new oral anticoagulants in critically ill patients, it is conceivable that a patient who is taking one of these agents may be admitted to the ICU, and therefore clinicians should be aware of the properties of these new drugs (**Table 3**). In particular, clinicians may be asked to deal with bleeding complications in patients taking these agents; this possibility is discussed in more depth later.

## USE OF ANTICOAGULANTS IN THE INTENSIVE CARE UNIT: PREVENTION OF VTE

VTE, which includes both DVT and PE, is a common cause of morbidity and mortality in critical care patients. Several studies illustrate the high incidence of VTE in ICU patients, many of whom are asymptomatic, despite aggressive use of thrombopro-phylaxis.[54–56] Critically ill medical and surgical patients pose a unique challenge to clinicians when using anticoagulants. These patients have a predilection for throm-bosis due to acquired risk factors including both the placement and presence of central venous catheters, other invasive procedures, mechanical ventilation with associated pharmacologic paralysis, prolonged immobilization, and acquired coag-ulation disorders. Also, low cardiac output and the use of vasopressors in this patient population may reduce the bioavailability of subcutaneous pharmacologic prophy-laxis.[57,58] Furthermore, ICU patients are at increased risk of bleeding because of acquired coagulopathies, thrombocytopenia or functional platelet disorders, drug interactions, recent surgeries or invasive procedures, and concomitant organ failure, especially of the liver or kidney. Therefore, a careful assessment of risks and benefits of prophylactic or therapeutic anticoagulation must be considered on an individual basis. Here the authors focus on the clinical trial evidence for VTE prophylaxis using the newer anticoagulants in critically ill patients.

Anticoagulant prophylaxis is the preferred approach in the prevention of VTE in medical-surgical ICU patients. Surveys of practice patterns, observational studies, and international registries indicate that clinicians most often prescribe UFH.[59–63] Within the last decade, adoption of LMWH prophylaxis has been explored because of high bioavailability, predictable anticoagulant effect, once-daily dosing, and studies showing lack of bioaccumulation in ICU patients with renal insufficiency.[64,65] Few studies have examined the safety and efficacy of LMWH in the ICU population. Although LMWH is more effective than UFH in trauma and spinal cord injury patients, the superiority of LMWH is debated in other ICU patients, as reflected in the 2012 ACCP guidelines.[54,66,67] Similarly, the Surviving Sepsis Campaign guidelines make Grade A recommendations (supported by at least two large randomized controlled trials with clear-cut results) for the use of thromboprophylaxis with either UFH or LMWH in severe sepsis patients.[68]

### LMWH Prophylaxis: Clinical Trial Evidence

To date, four randomized thromboprophylaxis trials and one metaanalysis have evaluated the safety and efficacy of LMWH either in comparison with placebo or UFH in critically ill patients (**Table 4**).[4,59,69–71] Whereas LMWH is superior to placebo[70] in ICU patients, whether this observation is more broadly applicable has been called into question by the recently published LIFENOX study in acutely ill medical patients.[72]

In a 2009 systematic review, Ribic and colleagues[59] accumulated data from eight observational studies and one randomized controlled trial, each of which examined the effect of LMWH thromboprophylaxis in medical-surgical critically ill pa-tients.[57,59,64,65,73–77] Studies that included only trauma or spinal cord injury patients

**Table 3**
Pharmacologic properties of the new oral anticoagulants

| Properties | Dabigatran | Rivaroxaban | Apixaban |
|---|---|---|---|
| Target | FIIa | FXa | FXa |
| Peak plasma concentrations | ~1.5 h | ~3 h | ~1–3 h |
| Half-life (normal Cr) | 12–14 h | 4–13 h | 8–15 h |
| Clearance | 80% renal | 60% renal | Multiple mechanisms |
| Antidote | No | No | No |
| Laboratory monitoring | Not required, TT/TCT or aPTT | Not required, anti-Xa assay | Not required, anti-Xa assay |
| Involvement of CYP | Minor | Minor | Minor |
| FDA indications | (1) Stroke and systemic embolism prophylaxis in nonvalvular atrial fibrillation | (1) VTE prophylaxis after TKR/THR (2) Stroke and systemic embolism prophylaxis in nonvalvular atrial fibrillation | None |

*Abbreviations:* Cr, creatinine; CYP, cytochrome p450; TKR, total knee replacement.

**Table 4**
Randomized controlled trials of LMWH for VTE prophylaxis in critical care patient

|  | Fraisse et al[69] | De et al[70] | Shorr et al (XPRESS)[71] | Cook et al (PROTECT)[4] |
|---|---|---|---|---|
| Patients (n) | 223 | 156 | 1935 | 3764 |
| Patient population | Mechanically ventilated for acute, decompensated COPD | Critically ill surgical patients undergoing major surgery | Severe sepsis requiring treatment with drotrecogin alfa | Critically ill patients in ICU |
| Groups | 1. Weight-adjusted nadroparin QD<br>2. Placebo | 1. UFH 5000 U BID<br>2. Enoxaparin 40 mg QD | 1. UFH 5000 U BID<br>2. Enoxaparin 40 mg QD<br>3. Placebo | 1. Dalteparin 5000 U QD<br>2. UFH 500 U BID |
| Primary efficacy outcome | DVT; nadroparin 15.5% vs placebo 28.2%, $P = .045$ | DVT: UFH 2.66% vs enoxaparin 1.23%, $P = .51$ | VTE: UFH 5.6%, enoxaparin 5.9%, placebo 7.0%, $P>.05$ | Proximal DVT: dalteparin 5.1% vs UFH 5.8%, $P = .57$ |
| Primary safety outcome | Overall hemorrhage: nadroparin 25% vs placebo 18%, $P = .18$ | Overall hemorrhage: UFH 24% vs 9.9%, $P = .01$<br>Major hemorrhage: UFH 2.66% vs 1.23% | NR | Major bleeding: dalteparin 5.5% vs UFH 5.6%, $P = .98$ |

Abbreviations: BID, twice daily; COPD, chronic obstructive pulmonary disease; NR, not reported; QD, daily.

were excluded given prior randomized controlled trials that had already established the superiority of LMWH in these patient populations. Various LMWH preparations and schedules were used in these studies. VTE in patients receiving LMWH ranged from 5.1% to 15.5%, bleeding complications from 7.2% to 23.1%, and mortality from 1.4% to 7.4%. The investigators concluded that LMWH cannot be recommended routinely in critically ill patients because no study had compared LMWH with an alternative thromboprophylaxis agent. Since the publication of this systematic review, three more randomized controlled trials have evaluated the use of LMWH prophylaxis in ICU patients.[69–71]

The efficacy and safety of nadroparin were compared with placebo in 223 patients mechanically ventilated for acute exacerbation of chronic obstructive pulmonary disease. Patients were randomized to treatment with weight-adjusted SQ nadroparin or placebo for an average duration of 11 days. DVT was significantly less frequent in patients receiving nadroparin compared with placebo (15.5% vs 28.2%, respectively; $P = .045$). There was no significant difference in hemorrhage between the two groups.[69]

In another trial, 156 critically ill patients anticipated to undergo major surgery within 24 hours were randomized to UFH 5000 units twice daily or enoxaparin 40 mg daily.[70] Major surgery was defined as any procedure under general anesthesia that was expected to take at least 1 hour and require at least 6 days hospitalization with at least 24 hours in the ICU. A critically ill patient was defined as demonstrating one or more organ failure requiring ICU monitoring for at least 24 hours. Prophylaxis was initiated within 12 hours preoperatively and continued for at least 6 days postoperatively. Doppler ultrasound of the lower extremities was performed for clinical suspicion of DVT as an inpatient, and for up to 6 months as outpatient. Baseline demographics were similar between the three groups. LMWH was as effective as UFH in the prophylaxis of DVT (1.23% vs 2.66%, respectively; $P = .51$). Major bleeding was similar between the two groups (2.66% vs 1.23%, respectively; $P = .48$). The investigators concluded that both UFH and LMWH prophylaxis are effective and safe for VTE prevention in critically ill surgical patients. Considering LMWH once-daily dosing, clinicians may prefer this mode of therapy to improve patient compliance and prevent medical errors because of missed doses. There is also some evidence that LMWH is associated with a lower risk of HIT.

In the XPRESS trial, patients with severe sepsis and higher disease severity who were being treated with drotrecogin alfa were randomized to enoxaparin 40 mg SQ daily, UFH 5000 units SQ twice daily, or placebo.[71] Doppler ultrasound of the lower extremities was performed for clinical symptoms suggestive of DVT and as surveillance between day 4 and day 6. At day 6, there was no statistically significant difference in any VTE event between the groups (UFH 5.0%, LMWH 4.2%, placebo 5.1%, $P>.05$). However, the study was underpowered to detect a difference between UFH and LMWH. Similar to others' observations, in this study most VTE events were clinically silent. Interestingly, less than half of patients were receiving pharmacologic prophylaxis prior to randomization, suggesting underutilization of VTE preventative strategies and lack of compliance with published guidelines in this high-risk ICU population.

In the PROTECT study, 3764 critically ill patients were randomly assigned to either dalteparin 5000 units SQ daily or UFH 5000 units SQ twice daily.[4] Dalteparin was selected as the comparator to UFH because of prior studies indicating lack of bioaccumlation in critically ill patients with a wide range of renal insufficiency.[64,65] The primary outcome, proximal leg DVT, was assessed by ultrasound of the lower extremities performed within 2 days of admission, twice weekly, and as clinically indicated. Major trauma, neurosurgery, or orthopedic surgery patients were excluded. The baseline characteristics of the two study groups were similar. No significant difference in proximal vein DVT was detected over the duration of ICU admission, which varied in length for individual patients (HR in favor of dalteparin .92; 95% CI .68–1.23; $P$ = .57). Clinically apparent PE was less frequent in the dalteparin group (HR .51; 95% CI .30–.88; $P$ = .01). The incidence of other secondary outcomes—any VTE, other DVT, or HIT—was no different between the groups. Major bleeding over the ICU stay occurred in 5.5% receiving dalteparin and 5.6% receiving UFH (HR 1.0; 95% CI .75—1.34, $P$ = .98)—despite the fact that patients allocated to either heparin or dalteparin could have any degree of renal impairment.

## SPECIAL CONSIDERATIONS IN ICU PATIENTS: POTENTIALS FOR OVERDOSING AND UNDERDOSING OF LMWH

Concerns about anticoagulant underdosing and overdosing in critically ill patients have been raised. Most of the data evaluating LMWH and VTE rates in the ICU population have reported anti-Xa measurements as a surrogate marker for LMWH anticoagulant effect, although this relationship remains to be validated. Although one advantage of LMWH is its predictable pharmacokinetics, certain characteristics of ICU patients such as organ dysfunction, impaired peripheral blood flow due to vasopressor use and low cardiac output, altered drug binding to albumin and acute phase reactants, and severe SQ edema may lead to changes in the absorption, distribution, metabolism, and clearance of the drug resulting in under- or overdosing.[57,78,79]

Because of the high incidence of renal impairment in ICU patients, studies have focused on detecting potential overdosing of LMWH in this population. For example, the DIRECT study evaluated 138 patients with a CrCl of less than 30 mL/min who received dalteparin 5000 units once daily. Bioaccumulation was defined as a trough anti-Xa level greater than .4I U/mL. Median duration of dalteparin exposure was 7 days. There was no evidence of bioaccumulation (0%; 95% CI 0–3.0%). Major bleeding occurred in 7.2% of patients (95% CI, 4.0%–12.8%) but could not be explained by LMWH adverse effect given low trough anti-Xa levels.[65] Rabbat and colleagues[64] studied 19 critically ill medical and surgical patients with renal insufficiency who received dalteparin 5000 units daily. They found no evidence of bioaccumulation of LMWH defined by trough anti-Xa levels. Furthermore, a correlation between clinical outcomes (bleeding and thrombosis) and LMWH anticoagulant effect as measured by anti-Xa levels could not be confirmed. In a single-dose observational study, Kani and colleagues[74] found that mean anti-Xa levels were comparable in patients with moderate (CrCl 30–50 mL/min) compared with those with severe (CrCl <30 mL/min) renal insufficiency. Whereas they found no evidence of bioaccumulation, these results are limited by the fact that bioaccumulation typically occurs only after multiple doses of LMWH.[74]

In contrast to potential for overdosing of LMWH, studies have reported low anti-Xa levels during critical illness.[79–82] Whether these low anti-Xa levels translate into higher thromboembolic events is controversial. Several prospective studies have revealed that standard doses of LMWH prophylaxis are ineffective in achieving recommended anti-Xa levels in ICU patients.[57,73,75,76] Risk factors that may correlate with low anti-Xa levels in ICU patients include multiple organ dysfunction, high body mass index, and vasopressor-induced peripheral vasoconstriction.[57,75,76] Severe subcutaneous edema from fluid resuscitation may impair absorption of various drugs used in the ICU. However, in a pilot study there was no clinically relevant difference in anti-Xa activity after SQ administration of dalteparin between medical-surgical ICU patients with and without subcutaneous edema. Dorffler-Melly and colleagues[77] showed that among patients who received at least 3 days of nadroparin thromboprophylaxis, the ICU patients receiving vasopressors had significantly lower systemic anti-Xa levels than other patients. These results raise the question of whether higher than usual prophylactic doses of LMWH are needed for adequate VTE prevention in certain ICU patients. The clinical significance of low anti-Xa levels in the surgical ICU after standard doses of LMWH prophylaxis was examined in a recent study.[75,76,80–82] Fifty-four patients received enoxaparin 30 mg SQ twice a day. Surveillance bilateral upper and lower extremity duplex ultrasounds were obtained within 48 hours of admission and then weekly thereafter. The primary outcome measure was occurrence of VTE. Fifty percent of patients had low anti-Xa levels, and this was associated with significantly more DVTs than those with normal levels (37% vs 11%, respectively; $P = .026$). No patient characteristics other than low peak anti-Xa levels were identified as potential predictors.

### Indirect Anti-Xa Inhibitors

No studies have evaluated the safety or efficacy of fondaparinux for VTE prevention in critically ill patients. In a multicenter prospective observational study, the bioavailability of fondaparinux in ICU patients with and without vasopressor requirements was assessed.[82] Among patients excluded were those with body mass index greater than 40 $kg/m^2$, CrCl at or below 30 mL/min, neuroaxial anesthesia or lumbar puncture, or liver failure. All patients received fondaparinux 2.5 mg SQ daily during the 5-day study period. A nonsignificant trend toward higher anti-Xa levels was found in the vasopressor group. The investigators concluded that vasopressor administration does not impair bioavailability of fondaparinux.

### New Oral Anticoagulants

To date, no data exist for the new oral anticoagulants (dabigatran, rivaroxaban, and apixaban) in the prevention of VTE in critically ill patients. Two studies have evaluated these agents in acute medical illness. The MAGELLAN study was a prospective, randomized, multinational clinical trial that included patients admitted for acute medical illness with at least one additional VTE risk factor. Patients were randomly assigned to receive either enoxaparin 40 mg SQ daily for 10 days or oral rivaroxaban 10 mg daily for 35 days. The primary efficacy outcome was asymptomatic proximal DVT, symptomatic DVT, symptomatic nonfatal PE, and VTE-related death. At 35 days, rivaroxaban was associated with a reduction in the risk of primary outcome (HR = .771, [95% CI .618–.962]; $P = .0211$). However, treatment-related major bleeding and clinically relevant nonmajor bleeding rates were significantly increased with rivaroxaban (RR = 2.5; $P<.0001$).[83]

The ADOPT study evaluated the efficacy and safety of prolonging VTE prophylaxis in medically ill patients beyond hospital discharge for a total of 30 days. High-risk medical patients hospitalized for congestive heart failure, acute respiratory failure, infection without septic shock, acute rheumatic disease, or inflammatory bowel disease and at least one additional VTE risk factor with anticipated hospital stay 3 days or longer were randomly assigned to apixaban 2.5 mg twice daily for 30 days or enoxaparin 40 mg SQ once daily for 6 to 14 days. Results indicated that extended prophylaxis with apixaban was not superior to shorter courses of enoxaparin in the prevention of VTE-related death, PE, symptomatic DVT, or asymptomatic proximal DVT at 30 days (RR .87; 95% CI, .62–1.23; $P = .44$). Apixaban was associated with significantly more major bleeding events than enoxaparin (RR 2.58; 95% CI, 1.02–7.24; $P = .04$).[84] Whether the results of the MAGELLAN and ADOPT study can be extrapolated to the ICU population remains to be seen. In the meantime, with long-term safety and efficacy data unknown, lack of antidote in bleeding scenarios, and effective alternative anticoagulants available, these new oral anticoagulants should be avoided in critically ill patients.

## MANAGEMENT OF BLEEDING

Bleeding is the primary complication of anticoagulation therapy.[85–87] Whereas reversal of older therapeutic agents such as UFH and warfarin is possible, many of the newer anticoagulants, including LMWHs, fondaparinux, DTIs, and the novel oral anticoagulants do not have a complete and specific antidote. Therefore the ideal method to manage bleeding with patients receiving these therapies is not known. Furthermore, accurate and widely available laboratory tests to measure anticoagulant activity may not be available for these newer agents.

Although protamine is a specific and effective reversal agent for UFH, it only neutralizes about 60% of LMWH's anticoagulant activity, and this degree varies based on the type of LMWH.[88] Adverse effects reported with protamine include allergic reactions, respiratory complications, hypotension, and bradycardia.[89] Fondaparinux is not reversed by protamine. In vitro studies and data from healthy volunteers suggest that recombinant factor VIIa (rFVIIa) may accelerate thrombin generation and normalize coagulation times in the presence of fondaparinux.[90,91]

Transfusion of fresh frozen plasma (FFP) in patients with anticoagulant-related bleeding should be reserved for those with a deficiency of coagulation factors (ie, resulting from vitamin K antagonists or dilutional coagulopathy) because FFP does not reverse anticoagulants that inhibit specific clotting factors. Clinicians should be aware of the potential for volume overload, transfusion related lung injury, and delays related to preparation and delivery of FFP.[92–94]

Although newer anticoagulants, including the factor X inhibitors (eg, fondaparinux, rivaroxaban, and apixaban) and the DTIs (eg, argatroban, bivalirudin, and dabigatran) have a shorter duration of anticoagulant effect than vitamin K antagonists, they do not have a true antidote. In the setting of life-threatening bleeding, rFVIIa may enhance thrombin generation and has been used off-label in the reversal of newer anticoagulants.[90,91]

Prothrombin complex concentrates (PCCs) are prepared from pooled plasma of many donors. PCCs are classified as 3-factor or 4-factor, depending on amount of vitamin K–dependent factors (II, VII, IX, X) that are included. 3- factor PCCs contain lower levels of factor VII and have traditionally been used to replace coagulation factors in patients with hemophilia B (factor IX deficiency); 4-factor PCCs have much larger amounts of factor VII and are more widely used to reverse anticoagulants. At the time of writing, no 4-factor PCCS were approved in the United States. No trials have compared the efficacy of 3-factor versus 4-factor PCCs. Three-factor PCCs may not correct the INR in warfarin-treated patients as effectively as 4-factor PCCs because of less FVII content. Whereas PCCs are typically used to reverse effects of warfarin therapy, they have also been suggested as adjunctive therapy in the treatment of bleeding related to the new oral anticoagulants.[92] However, when using rFVIIa or activated PCCs one must consider the potential thrombotic complications, especially in the hypercoagulable patient population that is normally using anticoagulant agents.

Desmopressin acetate (DDAVP) stimulates the release of factor VIII and von Willebrand factor from the endothelium into circulation. In vitro and animal models suggest that DDAVP may reduce the anticoagulant effect of lepirudin.[95–97] Side effects of DDAVP, a synthetic analog of vasopressin, include flushing, headaches, palpitations, hyponatremia, and tachyphylaxis. Tranexamic acid (Cyklokapron, Lysteda) and ε- aminocaproic acid (EACA; Amicar) block the proteolytic activity of plasmin and the conversion of plasminogen to plasmin, thereby stabilizing the fibrin clot. Use of these agents has been suggested to control anticoagulant bleeding due to DTIs.[85]

With any major anticoagulant-related bleeding, mechanical measures such as hemodialysis, hemofiltration, and plasmapheresis should be considered to physically remove anticoagulants from circulation. Addressing mechanical causes of bleeding may require radiologic, surgical, or endoscopic interventions. Acute hemodialysis may remove dabigatran because it has relatively low protein binding. More highly bound compounds, such as rivaroxaban and apixaban, are probably not removed with dialysis. Finally, supportive measures such as blood product transfusion, maintaining optimal body temperature, blood pH, electrolyte balance, and close surveillance of coagulation and hematologic parameters are essential as an adjunct to the previously described pharmacotherapy. Evidence-based guidelines are lacking, and most recommendations are based on anecdotal data and expert opinion. A summary of suggested recommendations for reversal of major bleeding with these newer agents is found in **Table 5**.

## PERIOPERATIVE INTERRUPTION OF ANTICOAGULATION

Interruption of anticoagulation before interventions with high risk of bleeding (eg, liver biopsy, surgery, neuroaxial anesthesia, and catheter insertion at noncompressible sites) must be weighed carefully against thrombotic risk. Renal and hepatic impairment, which can prolong clearance of anticoagulants, also need to be considered prior to discontinuation of the drug. Concomitant use of antiplatelet agents may exacerbate bleeding risk. The 2012 ACCP guidelines suggest in patients receiving therapeutic anticoagulation with LMWH to administer the last dose at 24 hours prior to surgery instead of 12 hours before surgery (Grade 2C).[99] The optimal time to discontinue fondaparinux preoperatively is less clear. With a half-life of 17 hours and even mild renal insufficiency prolonging clearance, therapeutic fondaparinux should be avoided in ICU patients who are expected to undergo invasive procedures.

Interruption of parenteral direct thrombin inhibitors such as bivalirudin, argatroban, and lepirudin should occur between 1 and 10 hours depending on degree of renal and hepatic impairment.[100] Normalization of the aPTT would indicate clearance of anticoagulant activity. Dabigatran should be discontinued at least 24 hours and up to 5 days prior to invasive procedure or surgery depending on degree of renal impairment and risk of bleeding.[37] Special considerations are taken in patients that require neuroaxial anesthesia as indicated by the recent American Society of Regional Anesthesia and Pain Medicine guidelines.[101] Black box warnings exist for patients on LMWH, fondaparinux, and rivaroxaban who are being considered for neuroaxial anesthesia,[10] although the increase in the risk of neuroaxial hematoma probably exists with any anticoagulant medication. Restarting anticoagulation in a timely manner postoperatively depends on individualized assessment of risks of bleeding from the procedure and thrombosis for underlying hypercoagulable state.

Postoperatively it is important to remember that, unlike warfarin, novel oral agents produce an essentially immediate therapeutic effect. Thus if patients are on agents such as dabigatran or rivaroxaban, and these drugs are interrupted for surgery, they should not be reintroduced until hemostasis is assured, probably several days after major or invasive surgery.

**Table 5**
Suggested recommendations for reversal of major bleeding on newer anticoagulants

| Anticoagulant | Reversal Agent | Dose/Timing | Laboratory Monitoring of Reversal | Special Considerations |
|---|---|---|---|---|
| LMWH<br>• Enoxaparin<br>• Dalteparin<br>• Tinzaparin | (1) Protamine<br>(2) rVIIa for life-threatening bleeding | (1) 1 mg protamine IV for each 1 mg of enoxaparin or 100 U of dalteparin tinzaparin given over prior 8 h.<br>(2) rVIIa 50–90 μg/kg IV. | Anti-Xa activity | Only partially reversed by protamine and may require repeated doses given half-life of LMWHs.<br>Protamine dose should be maintained <100 mg and administered slowly (≤5 mg/min). |
| Factor Xa inhibitor<br>• Fondaparinux<br>• Rivaroxaban<br>• Apixaban | (1) rVIIa | (1) No effective antidote. Poor quality evidence supports use of rVIIa in the case of truly life-threatening bleeding at a dose of 90 μg/kg IV. | Anti-Xa activity | Immediate effect.<br>Duration of effect 2–6 h.<br>Rivaroxaban: can use 50 U/kg IV PCC-based on 1 RCT in healthy subjects.[98] |
| Parenteral direct thrombin inhibitors<br>• Argatroban<br>• Lepirudin<br>• Bivalirudin<br>• Desirudin | (1) DDAVP<br>(2) Cryoprecipitate<br>(3) Antifibrinolytics | (1) DDAVP: .3 μg/kg.<br>(2) ≥10 U cryoppt.<br>(3) ε-aminocaproic acid (Amicar) .1–.15 g/kg IV over 30 min then infusion .5–1 g/h OR TXA 10 mg/kg IV q 6–8 h. | | DDAVP can be repeated q 8–12 h. Can develop tachyphylaxis, hyponatremia, and seizures. No more than two doses should be administered. |
| Oral direct thrombin inhibitor<br>• Dabigatran | (1) Oral charcoal<br>(2) rVIIa<br>(3) PCC | (1) Given within 2 h of last dose.<br>(2) rVIIa 60–90 μg/kg IV.<br>(3) PCC 25–100 U/kg IV depending on product used. | aPTT, TT/TCT | Consider HD especially if renal impairment. |

Insufficient data are available for formal evidence-based recommendations.
*Abbreviations:* HD, hemodialysis; q, every; RCT, randomized controlled trial; rFVIIa, recombinant factor VIIa; TXA, tranexamic acid.

## SUMMARY

VTE is a common complication of critical illness. Often DVT and PE are clinically silent and difficult to diagnose because of other comorbid conditions. Management and prevention of VTE in the critically ill patient can be complex and requires delicate consideration of the bleeding and thrombotic risks. Currently, UFH remains the standard of care for therapeutic anticoagulation in the ICU patient. LMWH is more effective than placebo and may be as effective as UFH in VTE prevention in this patient population. Other newer anticoagulants have yet to be studied rigorously in the ICU population and until then cannot be routinely recommended.

## REFERENCES

1. Garcia DA, Baglin TP, Weitz JI, et al. Parenteral anticoagulants: antithrombotic therapy and prevention of thrombosis, 9th ed: American College of Chest Physicians Evidence-Based Clinical Practice Guidelines. Chest 2012;141(2 Suppl):e24S–43S.
2. Hirsh J, Raschke R. Heparin and low-molecular weight heparin: the seventh ACCP Conference on Antithrombotic and Thrombolytic Therapy. Chest 2004;188S–203S.
3. Hawkins D, Evans J. Minimizing the risk of heparin-induced osteoporosis during pregnancy. Expert Opin Drug Saf 2005;4:583–90.
4. Cook D, Meade M, Guyatt G, et al. Dalteparin versus unfractionated heparin in critically ill patients. N Engl J Med 2011;364(14):1305–14.
5. Leizorovicz A, Siguret V, Mottier D. Safety profile of tinzaparin versus subcutaneous unfractioned heparin in elderly patients with impaired renal function treated for acute deep vein thrombosis: the Innohep in Renal Insufficiency Study (IRIS). Thromb Res 2011;128(1):27–34.
6. Lim W, Dentali F, Eikelboom J. Meta-analysis: low-molecular-weight heparin and bleeding in patients with severe renal insufficiency. Ann Intern Med 2006;144:673–84.
7. Weitz J, Middledorp S, Geerts W, et al. Thrombophilia and new anticoagulant drugs. Hematology Am Soc Hematol Educ Program 2004:424–38.
8. Weitz D, Weitz J. Update on heparin: what do we need to do? J Thromb Thrombolysis 2010;29:199–207.
9. Nagler M, Haslauer M, Wuillemin W. Fondaparinux - data on efficacy and safety in special situations. Thromb Res 2012;129(4):407–17.
10. US Department of Health and Human Services. US Food and Drug Administration. Available at: http://www.fda.gov. Accessed February 13, 2012.
11. Mehta SR, Boden WE, Eikelboom JW, et al. Antithrombotic therapy with fondaparinux in relation to interventional management strategy in patients with ST- and non-ST-segment elevation acute coronary syndromes: an individual patient-level combined analysis of the Fifth and Sixth Organization to Assess Strategies in Ischemic Syndromes (OASIS 5 and 6) randomized trials. Circulation 2008;118(25):e842.
12. Alban S. Pharmacological strategies for inhibition of thrombin activity. Curr Pharm Des 2008;14:1152–75.
13. Lewis B, Hursting M. Argatroban therapy in heparin-induced thrombocytopenia. In: Warkentin T, Greinacher A, editors. Heparin-induced thrombocytopenia. New York: Marcel Dekker; 2004. p. 437–74.
14. Williamson D, Boulanger I, Tardiff M. Argatroban dosing in intensive care patients with acute renal failure and liver dysfunction. Pharmacotherapy 2004;24:409–14.
15. Beiderlinden M, Treschan T, Gorlinger K, et al. Argatroban anticoagulants in critically ill patients. Ann Pharmacother 2007;41:749–54.
16. Lee C, Ansell J. Direct thrombin inhibitors. Br J Clin Pharmacol 2011;72:4, 581–92.

17. Hirsh J, Bauer KA, Donati MB, et al. Parenteral anticoagulants: American College of Chest Physicians evidence-based clinical practice guidelines (8th edition). Chest 2008;133(6 Suppl):141S–59S.
18. Nutescu EA, Shapiro NL, Chevalier A. New anticoagulant agents: direct thrombin inhibitors. Cardiol Clin 2008;26:169–87, v–vi.
19. Greinacher A, Warkentin TE. The direct thrombin inhibitor hirudin. Thromb Haemost 2008;99:819–29.
20. Celgene. Available at: http://www.celgene.com. Accessed February 13, 2012.
21. Nafziger AN, Bertino JS Jr. Desirudin dosing and monitoring in moderate renal impairment. J Clin Pharmacol 2010;50:614–22.
22. Iprivask [package insert]. Hunt Valley (MD): Canyon Pharmaceuticals, Inc; 2010.
23. Eriksson BI, Ekman S, Lindbratt S, et al. Prevention of thromboembolism with use of recombinant hirudin. Results of a double-blind, multicenter trial comparing the efficacy of desirudin (Revasc) with that of unfractionated heparin in patients having a total hip replacement. J Bone Joint Surg Am 1997;79:326–33.
24. Eriksson BI, Wille-Jorgensen P, Kalebo P, et al. A comparison of recombinant hirudin with a low-molecular-weight heparin to prevent thromboembolic complications after total hip replacement. N Engl J Med 1997;337:1329–35.
25. Antman EM. Hirudin in acute myocardial infarction. Thrombolysis and Thrombin Inhibition in Myocardial Infarction (TIMI) 9B trial. Circulation 1996;94(5):911–21.
26. The Global Use of Strategies to Open Occluded Coronary Arteries (GUSTO) IIb Investigators. A comparison of recombinant hirudin with heparin for the treatment of acute coronary syndromes. N Engl J Med 1996;335:775–82.
27. Rao K, Sun L, Chesebro JH, et al. Distinct effects of recombinant desulfatohirudin (Revasc) and heparin on plasma levels of fibrinopeptide A and prothrombin fragment F1.2 in unstable angina. A multicenter trial. Circulation 1996;94(10):2389–95.
28. Van Wyk V, Badenhorts PN, Luus HG, et al. A comparison between the use of recombinant hirudin and heparin during hemodialysis. Kidney Int 1995;48(4):1338–43.
29. Frame JN, Rice L, Bartholomew JR, et al. Rationale and design of the PREVENT-HIT study: a randomized, open-label pilot study to compare desirudin and argatroban in patients with suspected heparin-induced thrombocytopenia with or without thrombosis. Clin Ther 2010;32:626–36.
30. Bates SM, Weitz JI. The mechanism of action of thrombin inhibitors. J Invasive Cardiol 2000;12(Suppl F):27F–32.
31. Linkins L, Dans AL, Moores LK, et al. Treatment and prevention of heparin-induced thrombocytopenia: antithrombotic therapy and prevention of thrombosis, 9th ed: American College of Chest Physicians Evidence-Based Clinical Practice Guidelines Chest 2012;141(2 Suppl):e495S–530S.
32. Stangier J, Stahle H, Rathgen K. Pharmacokinetics and pharmacodynamics of the direct oral thrombin inhibitor dabigatran in healthy elderly subjects. Clin Pharmacokinet 2008;47(1):47–59.
33. Stangier J, Stahle H, Rathgen K, et al. Pharmacokinetics and pharmacodynamics of dabigatran etexilate, an oral direct thrombin inhibitor, are not affected by moderate hepatic impairment. J Clin Pharmacol 2008;48(12):1411–9.
34. Pradaxa [package insert]. Ridgefield (CT): Boehringer Ingelheim Pharmaceuticals; 2011.
35. Blech S, Ebner T, Ludwig-Schwellinger E, et al. The metabolism and disposition of the oral direct thrombin inhibitor, dabigatran, in humans. Drug Metab Dispos 2008;36(2):386–99.

36. Garcia D, Libby E, Crowther MA. The new oral anticoagulants. Blood 2010; 115(1):15–20.
37. Van Ryn J, Stangier J, Haertter S, et al. Dabigatran etexilate-a novel, reversible, oral direct thrombin inhibitor. Thromb Haemost 2010;103;1116–27.
38. Connolly SJ, Ezekowitz MD, Yusuf S, et al. Dabigatran versus warfarin in patients with atrial fibrillation. N Engl J Med 2009;361(12):1139–51.
39. Eriksson BI, Dahl OE, Rosencher N, et al. Oral dabigatran etexilate vs. subcutaneous enoxaparin for the prevention of venous thromboembolism after total knee replacement: the RE-MODEL randomized trial. J Thromb Haemost 2007;5(11):2178–85.
40. Eriksson BI, Dahl OE, Rosencer N, et al. Dabigatran etexilate versus enoxaparin for prevention of venous thromboembolism after total hip replacement: a randomized, double-blind, non inferiority trial. Lancet 2007;370(9591):949–56.
41. Schulman S, Kearon C, Kakkar AK, et al. Dabigatran versus warfarin in the treatment of acute venous thromboembolism. N Engl J Med 2009;361:2342–52.
42. Erikkson BI, Borris LC, Friedman RJ, et al. Rivaroxaban versus enoxaparin for thromboprophylaxis after hip arthroplasty. N Engl J Med 2008;358:2765–75.
43. Kakkar AK, Brenner B, Dahl OE, et al. Extended duration rivaroxaban versus short-term enoxaparin for the prevention of venous thromboembolism after total hip arthroplasty: a double-blind, randomized controlled trial. Lancet 2008;372:31–9.
44. Lassen MR, Ageno W, Borris LC, et al. Rivaroxaban versus enoxaparin for thromboprophylaxis after total knee arthroplasty. N Engl J Med 2008;358:2776–86.
45. Turpie AG, Lassen MR, Davidson BL, et al. Rivaroxaban versus enoxaparin for thromboprophylaxis after total knee arthroplasty (RECORD4): a randomised trial. Lancet 2009;373:1673–80.
46. Rocket Study Investigators. Rivaroxaban-once daily, oral, direct factor Xa inhibition compared with vitamin K antagonism for prevention of stroke and Embolism Trial in Atrial Fibrillation: rationale and design of the ROCKET AF study. Am Heart J 2010 2010;159(3):340–47, e1.
47. Weitz JI. Emerging anticoagulants for the treatment of venous thromboembolism. Thromb Haemost 2006;96 (3):274–84.
48. Eriksson BI, Dahl OE, Buller HR, et al. A new oral direct thrombin inhibitor, dabigatran etexilate, compared with enoxaparin for prevention of thromboembolic events following total hip or knee replacement: the BISTRO II randomized trial. J Thromb Haemost 2005;3:103–11.
49. Douketis J. Pharmacologic properties of the new oral anticoagulants: a clinician-oriented review with a focus on perioperative management. Curr Pharm Des 2010; 16:3436–41.
50. Eikelboom JW, Weitz JI. Dabigatran etexilate for prevention of venous thromboembolism. Thromb Haemost 2009;101:2–4.
51. Lassen M, Raskob G, Gallus A, et al. Apixaban or enoxaparin for thromboprophylaxis after knee replacement. N Engl J Med 2009;361:594–604.
52. Lassen M, Raskob G, Gallus A, et al. Apixaban versus enoxaparin for thromboprophylaxis after knee replacement (ADVANCE-2): a randomised double-blind trial. Lancet 2010;375:807–15.
53. Lassen MR, Gallus A, Raskob GE, et al. Apixaban versus enoxaparin for thromboprophylaxis after hip replacement. N Engl J Med 2010;363:2487–98.
54. Geerts WH, Jay RM, Code KI, et al. A comparison of low-dose heparin with low-molecular-weight heparin as prophylaxis against venous thromboembolism after major trauma. N Engl J Med 1996;335(10):701–7.
55. Hirsch DR, Ingenito EP, Goldhaber SZ. Prevalence of deep venous thrombosis among patients in medical intensive care. JAMA 1995;274(4):335–7.

56. Marik PE, Andrews L, Maini B. The incidence of deep venous thrombosis in ICU patients. Chest 1997;111:661–4.
57. Priglinger U, Delle Karth G, Geppert A, et al. Prophylactic anticoagulation with enoxaparin: is the subcutaneous route appropriate in the critically ill? Crit Care Med 2003;(5):1405–9.
58. Cook D, Crowther M, Meade M, et al. Deep venous thrombosis in medical-surgical critically ill patients: prevalence, incidence, and risk factors. Crit Care Med 2005; 33(7):1565–71.
59. Ribic C, Lim W, Cook D, et al. Low-molecular weight heparin thromboprophylaxis in medical-surgical critically ill patients: a systematic review. J Crit Care 2009;24(2): 197–205.
60. Cooper DJ, Bishop N, Cade J, et al. Australian and New Zealand Intensive Care Society Clinical Trials Group. Thromboprophylaxis for intensive care patients in Australia and New Zealand: a brief survey report. J Crit Care 2005;20(4):354–6.
61. Cook DJ, McMullin J, Hodder R, et al. for the Canadian ICU Directors Group. Prevention and diagnosis of venous thromboembolism in critically ill patients: a Canadian Survey. Crit Care 2001;5(6):336–42.
62. Cohen AT, Tapson VF, Bergmann JF, et al. Venous thromboembolism risk and prophylaxis in the acute hospital care setting (ENDORSE study): a multinational cross-sectional study. Lancet 2008;371:387–94.
63. Tapson VF, Decousus H, Pini M, et al. Venous thromboembolism prophylaxis in acutely ill medical patients: findings from the international medical prevention registry on venous thromboembolism (IMPROVE). Chest 1997;132:936–45.
64. Rabbat C, Cook D, Crowther M, et al. Dalteparin thromboprophylaxis for critically ill medical-surgical patients with renal insufficiency. J Crit Care 2005;20:357–63.
65. Douketis J, Cook D, Meade M, et al. Prophylaxis against deep vein thrombosis in critically ill patients with severe renal insufficiency with the low-molecular-weight heparin dalteparin. Arch Intern Med. 2008;168(16):1805–12.
66. Spinal Cord Injury Thromboprophylaxis Investigators. Prevention of venous thromboembolism and in the acute treatment phase after spinal cord injury: a randomized, multicenter trial comparing low-dose heparin plus intermittent pneumatic compression with enoxaparin. J Trauma 2003;54(6):116–24.
67. Kahn SR, Lim W, Dunn AS, et al. Prevention of VTE in nonsurgical patients: antithrombotic therapy and prevention of thrombosis, 9th ed: American College of Chest Physicians Evidence-Based Clinical Practice Guidelines. Chest 2012; 141(2 Suppl):e195S–226S.
68. Dellinger RP, Carlet JM, Masur H, et al. Surviving Sepsis Campaign guidelines for management of severe sepsis and septic shock. Crit Care Med 2004;32(3):858–73.
69. Fraisse F, Holzapfel L, Coulaud JM, et al. Nadroparin in the prevention of deep vein thrombosis in acute decompensated COPD. Am J Respir Crit Care Med 2000;161: 1109–14.
70. De A, Roy P, Garg VK, et al. Low-molecular-weight heparin and unfractionated heparin in prophylaxis against deep vein thrombosis in critically ill patients undergoing major surgery. Blood Coag Fibrinolysis 2010;21:57–61.
71. Shorr A, Williams M. Venous thromboembolism in critically ill patients. Thromb Haemost 2009;101:139–44.
72. Kakkar A, Cimminiello C, Goldhaber S, et al. Low-molecular-weight heparin and mortality in acutely ill medical patients. N Engl J Med 2011 365;26.
73. Rommers M, Van Der Lely N, Egberts T, et al. Anti-Xa activity after subcutaneous administration of dalteparin in ICU patients with and without subcutaneous oedema: a pilot study. Crit Care 2006;10:R93.

74. Kani C, Markantonis, S, Nicolaou C, et al. Monitoring of subcutaneous dalteparin in patients with renal insufficiency under intensive care: an observational study. J Crit Care 2006;21:79–84.

75. Jochberger S, Mayr V, Luckner G, et al. Antifactor Xa activity in critically ill patients receiving antithrombotic prophylaxis with standard dosages of certoparin: a prospective, clinical study. Crit Care 2005;9:R541–8.

76. Mayr AJ, Dunser M, Jochberger S, et al. Antifactor Xa activity in intensive care patients receiving thromboembolic prophylaxis with standard doses of enoxaparin. Thromb Res 2002;105:201–4.

77. Dorffler-Melly J, de Jonge E, de Pont AC, et al. Bioavailability of subcutaneous low-molecular-weight heparin to patients on vasopressors. Lancet 2002;359:849–50.

78. Krishnan V, Murray P. Pharmacologic issues in the critically ill. Clin Chest Med 2003;24:671–88.

79. Rutherford EJ, Schooler WG, Sredienski E, et al. Optimal dose of enoxaparin in critically ill trauma and surgical patients. J Trauma 2005;58:1167–70.

80. Haas CE, Nelsen JL, Raghavendran K, et al. Pharmacokinetics and pharmacodynamics of enoxaparin in multiple trauma patients. J Trauma 2005;59:1336–44.

81. Malinoski D, Jafari F, Ewing T, et al. Standard prophylactic enoxaparin dosing leads to inadequate anti-Xa levels and increased deep venous thrombosis rates in critically ill trauma and surgical patients. J Trauma 2012;68:874–80.

82. Cumbo-Nacheli G, Samavati L, Guzman J. Bioavailability of fondaparinux to critically ill patients. J Crit Care Med 2011;26:342–6.

83. Cohen AT, Sprio TE, Buller HR, et al. A rivaroxaban compared with enoxaparin for the prevention of venous thromboembolism in acutely ill medical patients [LBCT IV session 3015]. Presented at the ACC 60th Annual Scientific Sessions. New Orleans, LA, April 2–5, 2011.

84. Goldhaber S, Leizorovicz A, Kakkar A, et al. Apixaban versus enoxaparin for thromboprophylaxis in medically ill patients. N Engl J Med 365;23:2167–77.

85. Crowther M, Warkentin T. Bleeding risk and the management of bleeding complications in patients undergoing anticoagulant therapy: focus on new anticoagulant agents. Blood 2008;111:4871–9.

86. Levine MN, Raskob G, Beyth RJ, et al. Hemorrhagic complications of anticoagulant treatment: the Seventh ACCP Conference on Antithrombotic and Thrombolytic Therapy. Chest 2004;126;287S–310S.

87. Ng HJ, Crowther MA. New anti-thrombotic agents: emphasis on hemorrhagic complications and their management. Semin Hematol 2006;43:S77–83.

88. Crowther MA, Berry LR, Monagle PT, et al. Mechanisms responsible for the failure of protamine to inactivate low-molecular-weight heparin. Br J Haematol 2002;166:178–86.

89. Weiler JM, Gellhaus MA, Carter JG, et al. A prospective study of the risk of an immediate adverse reaction to protamine sulfate during cardiopulmonary bypass surgery. J Allergy Clin Immunol 1990;85:713–9.

90. Gerotziafas GT, Depasse F, Chakroun T, et al. Recombinant factor VIIa partially reverses the inhibitory effect of fondaparinux on thrombin generation after tissue factor activation in platelet rich plasma and whole blood. Thromb Haemost 2004;91:531–7.

91. Lisman T, Bigsterveld NR, Adelmeijer J, et al. Recombinant factor VIIa reverses the in vitro and ex vivo anticoagulant and profibrinolytic effects of fondaparinux. J Thromb Haemost 2003;1:2368–73.

92. Warkentin TE, Crowther MA. Reversing anticoagulants both old and new. Can J Anaesth 2002;49:S11–25.

93. Braunwald E, Antman EM, Beasley JW, et al. ACC/AHA 2002 guideline update for the management of patients with unstable angina and non-ST-segment elevation myocardial infarction-summary article: a report of the American College of Cardiology/American Heart Association task force on practice guidelines (Committee on the management of Patients with Unstable Angina). J Am Coll Cardiol 2004;44:E1–211.

94. Warkentin TE, Smith JW. The alloimmune thrombocytopenic syndromes. Transfus Med Rev 1997;11:296–307.

95. Ibbotson SH, Grant PJ, Kerry R, et al. The influence of infusions of 1-desamino-8-D-arginine vasopressin (DDAVP) in vivo on the anticoagulant effect of recombinant hirudin (CGP39393) in vitro. Thromb Haemost 1991;65:64–6.

96. Bove CM, Casey B, Marder VJ. DDAVP reduces bleeding during continued hirudin administration in the rabbit. Thromb Haemost 1996;75:471–5

97. Amin DM, Mant TG, Walker SM. Effect of a 15-minute infusion of DDAVP on the pharmacodynamics of REVASC during a four-hour intravenous infusion in healthy male volunteers. Thromb Haemost 1997;77:127–32.

98. Eerenberg ES, Kamphuisen PW, Sijpkens MK, et al. Reversal of rivaroxaban and dabigatran by prothrombin complex concentrates: a randomized, placebo controlled, crossover study in healthy subjects. Circulation 2011;124:1573–9.

99. Douketis JD, Spyropoulos AC, Spencer FA, et al. Perioperative management of antithrombotic therapy, 9th ed: American College of Chest Physicians Evidence-Based Clinical Practice Guidelines. Chest 2012;141(2 Suppl):e326S–50S.

100. Schaden E, Kozek-Langenecker SA. Direct thrombin inhibitors: pharmacology and application in intensive care medicine. Intensive Care Med 2010;36:1127–37.

101. Horlocker TT, Wedel DJ, Rowlingson JC, et al. Regional anesthesia in the patient receiving antithrombotic or thrombolytic therapy. American Society of Regional Anesthesia and Pain Medicine evidence-based guidelines (Third Edition). Reg Anesth Pain Med 2010;35:64–101.

# The Role of Plasmapheresis in Critical Illness

Trung C. Nguyen, MD[a,b,*], Joseph E. Kiss, MD[c], Jordana R. Goldman, MD[a], Joseph A. Carcillo, MD[d]

## KEYWORDS

- Therapeutic plasma exchange • Thrombotic microangiopathy
- Liver failure • Rapidly progressive glomerulonephritis • Vasculitides
- Solid organ transplantation

## KEY POINTS

- The American Society of Apheresis published a comprehensive evidence-based guideline to aid intensivists in using plasmapheresis as a therapeutic strategy.
- Plasmapheresis has seen an increase in usage in critically ill patients.
- Thrombotic microangiopathies, vasculitides, liver failure, ABO-incompatible solid organ transplantation, neurologic disorders, renal disorders, and immune dysregulation are some of the disorders in which intensivists could consider using plasmapheresis as a therapeutic strategy.

## INTRODUCTION

Since antiquity, mankind has hypothesized there are bad substances called "humors" that accumulate in the blood of sick patients and that the removal of these humors would make patients feel better. Bloodletting, the practice of draining blood from sick patients, has been around since the Egyptians, dating back 1000 years BC. The practice of bloodletting peaked in the 18th century and evolves with modern technology to this day. Blood has 4 major components: red blood cells, white blood cells, platelets, and plasma. With modern machinery, blood can be separated into each of these 4 components. Thus,

The authors have nothing to disclose.
[a] Section of Critical Care Medicine, Department of Pediatrics, Baylor College of Medicine/Texas Children's Hospital, 6621 Fannin, WT6-006, Houston, TX 77030, USA; [b] Division of Thrombosis Research, Department of Medicine, Baylor College of Medicine, Houston, TX 77030, USA; [c] The Institute of Transfusion Medicine, Division of Hematology/Oncology, Department of Medicine, University of Pittsburgh School of Medicine, Pittsburgh, PA 15220, USA; [d] Departments of Critical Care Medicine and Pediatrics, University of Pittsburgh School of Medicine, Pittsburgh, PA 15261, USA
* Section of Critical Care Medicine, Department of Pediatrics, Baylor College of Medicine/Texas Children's Hospital, 6621 Fannin, WT6-006, Houston, TX 77030.
*E-mail address:* tcnguyen@texaschildrenshospital.org

Crit Care Clin 28 (2012) 453–468
http://dx.doi.org/10.1016/j.ccc.2012.04.009
0749-0704/12/$ – see front matter © 2012 Elsevier Inc. All rights reserved.

if a particular blood component is causing harm, it can be selectively removed and replaced with the same blood component from healthy donors.

In this article, the authors will review the current recommendations from the American Society for Apheresis (ASFA) for plasmapheresis in many of the diseases that intensivists commonly encounter in critically ill patients.[1] Apheresis is derived from the Greek word *aphaeresis,* meaning "to take away." Plasmapheresis is an apheresis procedure that separates and removes the plasma component from a patient. Plasma exchange is when plasmapheresis is followed by replacement with fresh frozen plasma infusion.

## TECHNIQUES OF SEPARATING PLASMA FROM WHOLE BLOOD

Plasmapheresis is performed by 2 fundamentally different techniques: centrifugation or filtration. With centrifugation apheresis, whole blood is spun so that the 4 major blood components are separated out into layers by their different densities. With filtration plasmapheresis, whole blood passes through a filter to separate the plasma components from the larger cellular components of red blood cells, white blood cells, and platelets. Centrifugation apheresis is commonly performed by blood bankers. A major advantage is that there is no limit on the size of the molecules being removed. Its disadvantage is that it usually requires a consultation to another service such as a blood banker. Filtration plasmapheresis is commonly performed by nephrologists and intensivist. Its major advantage is that a large filter can be easily added to the existing continuous venovenous hemodialysis circuit without much interruption to patient care. However, a disadvantage is that the size of the molecules removed is limited by the size of the pore of the filter. This is problematic because certain plasma molecules are larger than existing available filters, for example the ultra-large von Willebrand factor multimers can measure up to 12 million daltons.

## PLASMAPHERESIS/PLASMA EXCHANGE IN CRITICALLY ILL PATIENTS

In 2010, ASFA published its updated comprehensive "Guidelines on the Use of Therapeutic Apheresis in Clinical Practice: Evidence-Based Approach From the Apheresis Applications Committee of the American Society for Apheresis."[1] The society divided its recommendations into 4 categories:

- **Category I:** "Disorder for which apheresis is accepted as first-line therapy, either as a primary standalone treatment or in conjunction with other modes of treatment."
- **Category II:** "Disorders for which apheresis is accepted as second-line therapy, either as a standalone treatment or in conjunction with other modes of treatment."
- **Category III:** "Optimum role of apheresis therapy is not established. Decision making should be individualized."
- **Category IV:** "Disorders in which published evidence demonstrates or suggests apheresis to be ineffective or harmful. Internal Review Board approval is desirable if apheresis treatment is undertaken in these circumstances."

This article reviews many of the diseases in critically ill patients that plasmapheresis/therapeutic plasma exchange (TPE) may play a role in the therapeutic strategy.

## THROMBOTIC MICROANGIOPATHIES

**Thrombotic microangiopathies** are syndromes associated with disseminated microvascular thrombosis.[2] Clinically, these syndromes manifest as new-onset thrombocytopenia and, if untreated, will lead to multiorgan failure and death. Thrombotic thrombocytopenic purpura (TTP), hemolytic uremic syndrome (HUS), disseminated intravascular coagulation (DIC), and catastrophic antiphospholipid syndrome (CAPS) are different spectrums of thrombotic microangiopathies. *"The ASFA gives a category I recommendation for plasmapheresis/therapeutic plasma exchange (TPE) in patients with TTP and atypical HUS due to autoantibody to factor H, category II recommendation for TPE in patients with CAPS, and a category III recommendation for TPE in patients with hematopoietic stem cell transplant–associated thrombotic microangiopathy."*[1]

## TTP

The classic "pentad" of TTP is thrombocytopenia, microangiopathic hemolytic anemia, neurologic abnormalities, renal failure, and fever. The underlying pathophysiologic process of TTP is the deficiency of ADAMTS-13 (aka, von Willebrand factor [VWF]–cleaving proteinase) leading to uncleaved thrombogenic large and ultra-large VWF.[2] Autopsies on patients who died from TTP demonstrate distinctive VWF- and platelet-rich microthrombi.[3–6] There are 2 forms of TTP: congenital and acquired. In the congenital form, there is a genetic abnormality in ADAMTS-13.[7] In the acquired form, ADAMTS-13 inhibitors and/or proteolytic inactivators are present in the plasma.[8,9] There is a growing list of ADAMTS-13 inhibitors and proteolytic inactivators including interleukin-6, plasma-free hemoglobin, IgG autoantibody, *Shiga* toxin, plasmin, thrombin, and granulocyte elastase.[9–14] TPE has been shown in a large randomized controlled trial to significantly improve survival compared to plasma infusion.[15] The *ASFA gives a category I recommendation for TPE in TTP.*[1]

TPE is thought to remove the large and ultra-large VWF, remove the ADAMTS-13 inhibitors and proteolytic inactivators, and replenish ADAMTS-13.[2] Because the underlying pathology is the deficiency of ADAMTS-13, the recommended TPE replacement fluid is plasma or plasma with cryoprecipitate removed (ie, the plasma portion that is depleted with ultra-large VWF and large plasma VWF).

## Typical HUS

The "triad" of HUS is thrombocytopenia, microangiopathic hemolytic anemia, and renal failure.[2] This syndrome is divided into typical HUS and atypical HUS. Typical HUS, which accounts for 85% to 90% of all HUS, is commonly associated with infection and diarrhea.[16,17] *Shiga* toxin–producing *Escherichia coli* O157:H7 accounts for the majority of typical HUS with a mortality of less than 5%. *Shiga* toxin has been shown in vitro to (1) induce ultra-large VWF to be released from endothelium and (2) inhibit ADAMTS-13, similar to the pathophysiology of TTP. However, clinical association studies have not consistently shown severe ADAMTS-13 deficiency in *E coli* O157:H7–induced HUS.[6] Certain neuramidase producing-bacteria, such as *Streptococcus pneumoniae*, account for a minority of typical HUS cases and has a higher mortality compared to that of typical HUS with a mortality rate of 19% to 50%. Neuramidase has been shown to cleave sialic acid residues from cell surface protein exposing the Thomsen-Freidenreich (T-) antigen. HUS occurs when endogenous IgM directed against the T-antigen binds to the exposed T-antigen on endothelium, red blood cells, and platelets resulting in platelet-rich thrombi formation in the microvasculature. Currently, the *ASFA does not recommend TPE (category IV) for typical HUS.*[1]

## Atypical HUS

In atypical HUS, in addition to the typical "triad" of signs and symptoms, patients have neurologic abnormalities beyond that of the usual "irritability" seen in most children with typical HUS. Investigation into pathophysiology of atypical HUS has identified 2 different processes: genetic abnormalities or acquired autoantibodies. Currently, it is thought that up to 60% of patients with atypical HUS have genetic abnormalities in the complement pathway.[17] Autoantibodies against factor H have been observed in up to 10% of patients with atypical HUS.[17] In either case, there is uncontrolled activation of the alternative complement pathway, resulting in direct injury to the microvasculature. Atypical HUS has a reported mortality rate of 25%.[17]

*The ASFA gives a category I recommendation for TPE in atypical HUS due to autoantibody to factor H.*[1] Factor H regulates and inhibits the alternative pathway of the complement pathway. TPE is thought to remove the autoantibody to factor H and normalize complement activities.[18]

*The ASFA gives a category II recommendation for TPE in atypical HUS due to complement factor gene mutations.*[1] These genes include inhibitors of alternative complement pathways such as factor H, factor I, membrane cofactor protein, complement factor H–related proteins, and C4b binding protein. Gain-of-function mutations for alternative complement pathways also been described such as factor B and C3.[17]

During the first 24 to 72 hours of a patient presenting with the "triad" of signs and symptoms, along with neurologic abnormalities, most clinicians are not able to differentiate TTP from atypical HUS or differentiate atypical HUS due to autoantibody to factor H from atypical HUS as a result of complement factor gene mutations. We recommend consulting nephrology and hematology to send the appropriate ADAMTS-13, VWF, and complement studies. In addition, TPE should be initiated until the results of biomarkers can differentiate the diagnoses. Because the underlying pathology is the deficiency of complement H activity, the recommended TPE replacement fluid is either plasma or albumin. We recommend plasma as the replacement fluid since it has normal factor H activity.

## DIC

DIC is characterized by intravascular activation of coagulation leading to the consumption and exhaustion of coagulation proteins and platelets. Autopsies in patients who died with DIC reveal extensive fibrin deposition in small and middle-sized vessels in all organs.[3,4,6,19] One of the proposed mechanisms for DIC is that systemic inflammation, such as occurs in sepsis, activates leukocytes and endothelium. These cells then synthesize, express, and release tissue factor. Tissue factor forms a complex with factor VII, leading to the activation of coagulation and the resultant disseminated microvascular thrombosis with fibrin-rich microthrombi.[20] Clinically, these patients present with shock and in a prothrombotic and antifibrinolytic state with subsequent bleeding diathesis. Many case series and observational studies suggest that TPE might have a beneficial effect in DIC.[21-25] TPE is thought to normalize the blood coagulation to homeostasis milieu by removing tissue factor and plasminogen activator inhibitors type I and by replacing antithrombin III, protein C, and coagulation factors. Currently, the ASFA does not have a specific recommendation for TPE in DIC.

However, *the ASFA gives a category III recommendation for TPE in sepsis with multiorgan failure.*[1] Large trials have documented that sepsis can induce thrombotic microangiopathy, and, in particular, sepsis-induced DIC is present in 30% to 50% of patients with severe sepsis.[19,26] DIC has been shown to be one of the major contributing mechanisms to multiorgan failure in critically ill patients.[19] Thus, there is a biologic plausibility that the beneficial treatment effect of TPE in *sepsis with multiorgan failure* could be from reversing DIC.

### Thrombocytopenia-Associated Multiple Organ Failure

Recently, investigators observed that pediatric patients with thrombocytopenia-associated multiorgan failure (TAMOF) have thrombotic microangiopathy and that TPE may have a beneficial effect.[25] These investigators reported that pediatric patients with new-onset thrombocytopenia defined as platelet counts less than 100,000/mm$^3$ and at least 3 failing organs have a pathophysiologic process similar to that of TTP such as low ADAMTS-13 activities, presence of ultra-large VWF, and high VWF activities. A subset of TAMOF patients also had prolonged prothrombin time suggesting fibrin pathway activation, as in DIC. On autopsies, pediatric TAMOF patients have VWF-rich and platelet-rich microthrombi similar to patients with TTP and also fibrin-rich microthrombi similar to patients with DIC. In a small single-center trial, they reported that TPE had a significant beneficial treatment effect in reducing organ failure score (pediatric logistic organ dysfunction) and mortality. Of note, all of these patients had concurrent sepsis. Thus, *the ASFA category III recommendation for TPE in sepsis with multiorgan failure,*[1] as discussed earlier, encompasses sepsis-induced TAMOF.

A larger multicenter registry of TPE in pediatric TAMOF is in its analysis phase. Hopefully, this registry will shed more light on the treatment effect of TPE for TAMOF. Because the underlying pathology could be in part from deficient coagulation factors due to consumption, the recommended TPE replacement fluid is either plasma or albumin. The authors recommend plasma as the replacement fluid.

### CAPS

The underlying pathology in CAPS is an acquired hypercoagulable state due to the presence of antiphospholipid, anticardiolipin, and/or anti-beta 2 glycoprotein I antibodies.[27] The clinical presentation is acute microvascular venous and arterial thrombosis leading to multiorgan failure. Currently, the definition of CAPS includes (1) involvement of at least 3 organs, (2) manifestation in less than 1 week, (3) confirmed histopathology of small vessel occlusion in 1 tissue, and (4) presence of antiphospholipid antibodies.[28] This syndrome may be clinically indistinguishable from TTP, HUS, DIC, and TAMOF. For example, overt DIC is present in 20% of patients with CAPS. Biomarkers could help to differentiate between CAPS from TTP, HUS, and DIC.

*The ASFA gives a category II recommendation for TPE in CAPS.*[1] TPE is thought to remove antiphospholipid antibodies, inflammatory cytokines, and complement and to replace the deficient coagulation factors.[29–31] The recommended TPE replacement fluid is plasma as it has normal level of coagulation proteases.

### Hematopoietic Stem Cell Transplant–Associated Thrombotic Microangiopathy

The causes of thrombotic microangiopathy in hematopoietic stem cell transplant are unclear.[32–35] Endotheliopathy is suggested to be the underlying pathophysiologic process.[36] However, it is postulated that there could be multiple triggers including high-dose conditioning chemotherapy, irradiation, graft-versus-host disease, mammalian target of rapamycin, and calcineurin inhibitor drugs, as well as infection. The mainstay of therapy involves treating graft-versus-host disease, reducing doses of the mammalian target of rapamycin and calcineurin inhibitor drugs, and treating infection. ADAMTS-13 activities have been shown to be low-normal in these patients. Some patients seem to respond to TPE. Thus, a trial of TPE with a defined endpoint in selected patients with persistent thrombotic microangiopathy might be considered.[37–39]

*The ASFA gives a category III recommendation for TPE in hematopoietic stem cell transplant–associated thrombotic microangiopathy.[1] The recommended TPE replacement fluid is plasma or plasma with cryoprecipitate removed.*

### Thrombotic Microangiopathy: Drug-Associated

A number of drugs have been shown to activate platelets and/or cause endotheliopathy. Antiplatelet drugs such as ticlopidine and clopidogrel are members of the thienopyridine class of drugs that inhibit the adenosine diphosphate receptor/P2Y12 on platelets. They have been shown to induce TTP-like pathophysiology with low ADAMTS-13 activities and clinical signs of thrombotic microangiopathy in rare cases.[40–42] Calcineurin inhibitors such as cyclosporine and tacrolimus have been reported to induce endotheliopathy, progressing to thrombotic microangiopathy.[43–46] Management includes either stopping the offending drug or, if this is not an option, at least reducing the drug intake. TPE is thought to be beneficial similar to its use in acquired TTP.

*The ASFA gives a category I recommendation for TPE in ticlopedine or clopidogrel and a category III recommendation for TPE in cyclosporine- or tacrolimus-associated thrombotic microangiopathy.[1] The recommended TPE replacement fluid is plasma or plasma with cryoprecipitate removed.*

## VASCULITIDES
### CAPS

This syndrome is often grouped with vasculitides as it is diagnosed by rheumatologists. However, CAPS is a thrombotic microangiopathy and has significant overlap with TTP, HUS, DIC, and TAMOF. (Please refer to the earlier discussion in Thrombotic Microangiopathies for a review of CAPS.)

### Systemic Lupus Erythematosus

Systemic lupus erythematosus (SLE) is an autoimmune disorder that causes chronic inflammation due to circulating autoantibodies, immune complexes, and complement deposition. SLE is much more common in women than in men. Clinical symptoms such as malaise, arthritis, rash, and fever are nonspecific and often vary from person to person. However, severe progression of disease can occur with involvement of virtually any organ with consequent manifestations such as stroke, renal failure, pulmonary hemorrhage, myocarditis, hemolytic anemia, and pulmonary embolism. Confirmatory tests include the presence of specific antinuclear antibodies such as anti–double-stranded DNA and anti-Smith antibodies. First-line therapy includes anti-inflammatory and immunosuppressive agents. However, when severe SLE presents with cerebritis or pulmonary hemorrhage, TPE is recommended.[47–50]

*The ASFA gives a category II recommendation for TPE in severe SLE such as with cerebritis or diffuse alveolar hemorrhage.[1]* The ASFA does not recommend TPE (category IV) for SLE-associated nephritis. TPE is thought to remove autoantibodies, complement, interferon alpha, and immune complexes.[51,52] The recommended TPE replacement fluid is either plasma or albumin.

## LIVER FAILURE
### Wilson's Disease in Fulminant Hepatic Failure with Hemolysis

Wilson's disease is an autosomal recessive genetic disorder that results in excessive accumulation of copper in the liver, brain, cornea, kidney, and heart.[53] The genetic mutation is on the *ATP7B* gene, which codes for P-type ATPase (cation transport enzyme). This leads to impaired biliary copper excretion and linkage of copper to ceruloplasmin, a copper-carrying protein. As copper continues to accumulate in the liver, patients may present with asymptomatic elevation of liver enzymes, hepatitis, cirrhosis, or fulminant liver failure. These patients may also present with hemolytic anemia due to copper-induced oxidative stress to red blood cell enzymatic metabolic pathways or direct damage to the cell membrane. When patients with Wilson's disease present with fulminant liver failure, it is thought that a significant amount of copper is released from necrotic hepatocytes. Plasma-free copper then causes rapid destruction of red cells, which leads to rapid release of plasma-free hemoglobin. Elevated plasma-free hemoglobin has been shown to cause oxidative stress, nitric oxide depletion, endotheliopathy, microvascular thrombosis, and multiorgan failure. The only definite therapy is liver transplantation. However, without aggressive support, the patient is at risk of dying before liver transplantation.

The ASFA gives a category I recommendation for TPE in fulminant hepatic failure with hemolysis.[1] TPE is thought to provide rapid removal of plasma-free copper and hemoglobin.[54–58] The recommended TPE replacement fluid is plasma.

### Acute Fulminant Liver Failure

Acute fulminant liver failure has many causes and can develop from previously healthy liver or from chronic liver failure.[59] The liver has 4 major functions: protein synthesis, toxin clearance, gluconeogenesis/glycolysis, and biliary clearance. When the functions of protein synthesis and toxin clearance are severely compromised, severe clinical deterioration ensues. The liver synthesizes most of the major coagulation proteases. Without these, patients may develop severe coagulopathy and are at high risk of spontaneous hemorrhages, especially in the brain. In addition, patients are also at high risk for developing severe cerebral edema due to accumulation of toxins such as ammonia, endogenous benzodiazepines, and aromatic amino acids, among others.[60,61] If there is no spontaneous recovery of liver function, patients will require liver transplantation. Currently, there are no U.S. Food and Drug Administration–approved liver-support devices. Clinicians are only able to provide supportive care for these patients such as transfusion of blood products, securing the airway for hepatic coma, providing medical support for increased intracranial pressure, providing hemodynamic support, and appropriate antibiotics. These strategies, however, do not address the accumulation of toxins in the plasma. Furthermore, large amount of blood product transfusions and the commonly associated hepatorenal syndrome will inevitably lead to severe fluid overload. TPE is thought to remove the accumulation of toxins in the plasma and to restore coagulation back to its homeostasis milieu without fluid overloading the patients.[60,62–64]

The ASFA gives a category III recommendation for TPE in acute liver failure.[1] The recommended TPE replacement fluid is plasma or mixed plasma and albumin.

## SOLID ORGAN TRANSPLANTATIONS
### ABO-Incompatible Solid Organ Transplantation

Due to shortage of available organs and especially ABO-matched organs, ABO-incompatible organs are now frequently used in transplantation. During and after an ABO-incompatible solid organ transplantation, the recipient's natural antibodies to the A and/or B antigen on the donated organ will start to cause destruction of the newly grafted organ.[65] This might present as a hyperacute or acute humoral rejection. The mainstay of therapy has been immunosuppression. However, with the adjunct of TPE during the pre- and post-transplantation periods, along with immunosuppression and intravenous immunoglobulin (IVIG), survival of ABO-incompatible organs is comparable to those of ABO-matched organs.

The ASFA gives a category II recommendation for TPE in ABO-incompatible heart (<40 months of age) and kidney and a category III recommendation for ABO-incompatible liver (liver perioperative).[1] The goal is to decrease the IgG and IgM titers to 8 or less in liver and less than 4 in kidney and heart transplantations.[66–68] For liver transplants, an antibody titer of less than 8 should be aimed for 2 weeks post-transplant. For kidney transplants, the goal should be an antibody titer of less than 8 during the first week and less than 16 during the second week.[69,70] The recommended TPE replacement fluid is either albumin or plasma. For liver transplantation, plasma should be considered if there is significant coagulopathy.

## NEUROLOGIC DISORDERS

The ASFA gives strong recommendations (categories I and II) for TPE in critically ill patients with a variety of primary neurologic disorders.[1] The proposed mechanism of these disorders seems to stem from molecules (ie, autoantibodies) that have developed in the patient's plasma that cause injuries to the central and/or peripheral nervous systems. These patients often present with focal neurologic deficits and may progress to generalized devastating neurologic injuries. For example, these patients may present with gross or fine motor weakness progressing to paralysis, hyporeflexia progressing to areflexia, paresthesia, pain, cranial nerve deficit, seizures, strokes, autonomic dysfunction, and neuropsychiatric symptoms. TPE is often used by the clinicians when a short trial of steroids, cytotoxic agents, and/or IVIG has been unsuccessful in halting the progression of signs and symptoms.[71–75]

The ASFA gives a category I recommendation for TPE in acute inflammatory demyelinating polyneuropathy (Guillain-Barre syndrome), chronic inflammatory demyelinating polyradiculoneuropathy, pediatric autoimmune neuropsychiatric disorders associated with streptococcal infections and Sydenham's chorea, multiple sclerosis, and myasthenia gravis. The ASFA gives a category II recommendation for TPE in acute disseminated encephalomyelitis, neuromyelitis optica, chronic focal encephalitis (Rasmussen's encephalitis), and Lambert-Eaton myasthenic syndrome.[1]

TPE is thought to remove autoantibodies to various components of the neurologic system:

- Myelin in Guillain-Barre, chronic inflammatory demyelinating polyradiculoneuropathy, multiple sclerosis, and acute disseminated encephalomyelitis
- Neurons in the basal ganglia in pediatric autoimmune neuropsychiatric disorders associated with streptococcal infections and Sydenham's chorea
- Acetylcholine receptor on the postsynaptic surface of the motor end plate in myasthenia gravis
- Aquaporin-4, a water channel on astrocyte foot process at the blood-brain barrier in neuromyelitis optica
- Glutamate receptor GluR3 in Rasmussen's encephalitis
- Voltage-gated calcium channel of the presynaptic neuron in Lambert-Eaton myasthenic syndrome.[71,74,76,77]

Because the underlying problem is the presence of pathologic autoantibodies and not the deficiency of plasma molecules, the recommended TPE replacement fluid is albumin.

## RENAL
### Rapidly Progressive Glomerulonephritis

Rapidly progressive clomerulonephritis (RPGN) encompasses 3 distinct histopathologic processes of glomerular crescent formation in at least 50% of glomeruli seen in renal biopsies. Clinically, these patients might present with a rapid course of renal failure. Therapy involves a combination of steroids and anticytotoxic agents. TPE is considered when these patients present critically ill and, in particular, with pulmonary hemorrhage. The recommendation for TPE is also dependent on the histopathologic process.

### Type I RPGN: anti–glomerular basement membrane disease (goodpasture's syndrome)

Histopathology of this entity reveals linear deposits of IgG to the noncollagenous domain of the alpha-3 chain of collagen type IV in the glomerular basement membrane. *The ASFA gives a category I recommendation for TPE in anti–glomerular basement membrane disease with diffuse alveolar hemorrhage and/or with dialysis independence.*[1] The ASFA does not recommend (category IV) TPE for this entity with dialysis dependence and without diffuse alveolar hemorrhage.[1] Case series have shown that TPE in those with creatinine less than 6.6 mg/dL had recovery of kidney function, whereas those with creatinine greater than 6.6 mg/dL did not. The recommended TPE replacement fluid is albumin, but if pulmonary hemorrhage is present, then plasma is recommended.[78–81]

### Type II RPGN: immune complex rapidly progressive glomerulonephritis

Histopathology of this entity reveals granular deposits of immune complexes from a wide range of causes including post-streptococcal glomerulonephritis, membranoproliferative glomerulonephritis, lupus nephritis, IgA nephropathy, and Henoch-Schonlein purpura.[82,83] *The ASFA gives a category III recommendation for TPE in immune complex RPGN.*[1] The recommended TPE replacement fluid is albumin.

### Type III RPGN: anti–neutrophil cytoplasmic antibodies (ANCA)–associated RPGN (wegener's granulomatosis)

Histopathology of this entity reveals minimal immune deposits in the glomerulus. However, the serum contains the distinctive biomarker ANCA. *The ASFA gives a category I recommendation for TPE in ANCA-associated RPGN with diffuse alveolar hemorrhage and/or with dialysis dependence and a category III for those with dialysis independence.*[1] The recommended TPE replacement fluid is albumin but, if pulmonary hemorrhage is present, then plasma is recommended.[84–87]

## OTHER CONDITIONS
### Hemophagocytic Lymphohistiocytosis: Pathologic Hyperactive Inflammation

Secondary hemophagocytic lymphohistiocytosis (HLH) has been increasingly diagnosed in the intensive care unit. HLH is a syndrome of pathologic hyperactive inflammation due to unchecked immune activation.[88] Primary HLH is associated with genetic mutations such as those in the perforin gene. Perforin is normally secreted from cytotoxic T-lymphocytes and natural killer cells into the membrane of target cells and acts to trigger cell death. HLH occurs when lymphocyte-mediated cytotoxicity is impaired and apoptosis is unable to be triggered. This leads to abnormal T-cell activation and pathologic inflammatory cytokine production. Clinically these patients progress to multiorgan failure with the following clinical criteria: (1) fever; (2) splenomegaly; (3) cytopenia; (4) hypertriglyceridemia; (5) hemophagocytosis in bone marrow, spleen, lymph nodes, or liver; (6) low or absent NK-cell activity; (7) ferritin greater than 500 ng/mL, and (8) elevated serum CD 25 (alpha-chain of soluble interleukin-2 receptor).[88,89] The primary treatment for familial/primary HLH is a course of immunosuppression and bone marrow transplantation. Secondary HLH is an acquired form of pathologic hyperactive inflammation due to a trigger. Epstein-Barr virus is the most commonly recognized infection associated with secondary HLH. For other associated viral, bacterial, and fungal infections, the line between secondary HLH and sepsis-induced multiorgan failure due to other mechanisms, such as immune paralysis with unresolved infection and thrombotic microangiopathy, is blurred.[90] Much research is still needed to define the best strategy to balance the immune modulation. Too much immunosuppression in an immune paralyzed patient with unresolved infection could be detrimental. Inadequate immunosuppression in an uncontrolled pathologic hyperactive inflammation (ie, secondary HLH) could also be detrimental.

TPE has been reported in many small case series to be beneficial in calming the cytokine storm and to provide hematologic support in patients with primary and secondary HLH.[91–99] A recent small study found significant improved survival in patients with secondary HLH who received plasma exchange, steroids, and IVIG (n = 17) versus those who received plasma exchange, steroids, and/or cyclosporine, and/or etoposide (n = 6).[100] Currently, the ASFA has not commented on the use of TPE in HLH. Further research is warranted for this difficult therapeutic strategy.

## SUMMARY

TPE is a modern approach to the ancient therapy of bloodletting. Recently, the ASFA, using an evidence-based approach, published a comprehensive apheresis guideline to aid physicians caring for critically ill patients who depend on plasmapheresis as a therapeutic strategy. We are indebted to them for their hard work. It seems that TPE as a therapy has seen an increase in use, particularly by those who take care of critically ill patients. Using an evidence-based approach is the best way to standardize care and to provide a platform for innovation to move the field forward.

## REFERENCES

1. Szczepiorkowski ZM, Winters JL, Bandarenko N, et al. Guidelines on the use of therapeutic apheresis in clinical practice: evidence-based approach from the Apheresis Applications Committee of the American Society for Apheresis. J Clin Apher 2010;25(3):83–177.
2. Moake JL. Thrombotic microangiopathies. N Engl J Med 2002;347(8):589–600.
3. Asada Y, Sumiyoshi A, Hayashi T, et al. Immunohistochemistry of vascular lesion in thrombotic thrombocytopenic purpura, with special reference to factor VIII related antigen. Thromb Res 1985;38(5):469–79.
4. Burke AP, Mont E, Kolodgie F, et al. Thrombotic thrombocytopenic purpura causing rapid unexpected death: value of CD61 immunohistochemical staining in diagnosis. Cardiovasc Pathol 2005;14(3):150–5.
5. Hosler GA, Cusumano AM, Hutchins GM. Thrombotic thrombocytopenic purpura and hemolytic uremic syndrome are distinct pathologic entities. A review of 56 autopsy cases. Arch Pathol Lab Med 2003;127(7):834–9.
6. Tsai HM, Chandler WL, Sarode R, et al. von Willebrand factor and von Willebrand factor-cleaving metalloprotease activity in Escherichia coli O157:H7-associated hemolytic uremic syndrome. Pediatr Res 2001;49(5):653–9.
7. Levy GG, Nichols WC, Lian EC, et al. Mutations in a member of the ADAMTS gene family cause thrombotic thrombocytopenic purpura. Nature 2001;413(6855): 488–94.

8. Furlan M, Robles R, Galbusera M, et al. von Willebrand factor-cleaving protease in thrombotic thrombocytopenic purpura and the hemolytic-uremic syndrome. N Engl J Med 1998;339(22):1578–84.

9. Tsai HM, Lian EC. Antibodies to von Willebrand factor-cleaving protease in acute thrombotic thrombocytopenic purpura. N Engl J Med 1998;339(22):1585–94.

10. Bernardo A, Ball C, Nolasco L, et al. Effects of inflammatory cytokines on the release and cleavage of the endothelial cell-derived ultralarge von Willebrand factor multimers under flow. Blood 2004;104(1):100–6.

11. Crawley JT, Lam JK, Rance JB, et al. Proteolytic inactivation of ADAMTS13 by thrombin and plasmin. Blood 2005;105(3):1085–93.

12. Studt JD, Hovinga JA, Antoine G, et al. Fatal congenital thrombotic thrombocytopenic purpura with apparent ADAMTS13 inhibitor: in vitro inhibition of ADAMTS13 activity by hemoglobin. Blood 2005;105(2):542–4.

13. Nolasco LH, Turner NA, Bernardo A, et al. Hemolytic uremic syndrome-associated Shiga toxins promote endothelial-cell secretion and impair ADAMTS13 cleavage of unusually large von Willebrand factor multimers. Blood 2005;106(13):4199–209.

14. Ono T, Mimuro J, Madoiwa S, et al. Severe secondary deficiency of von Willebrand factor-cleaving protease (ADAMTS13) in patients with sepsis-induced disseminated intravascular coagulation: its correlation with development of renal failure. Blood 2006;107(2):528–34.

15. Rock GA, Shumak KH, Buskard NA, et al. Comparison of plasma exchange with plasma infusion in the treatment of thrombotic thrombocytopenic purpura. Canadian Apheresis Study Group. N Engl J Med 1991;325(6):393–7.

16. Delvaeye M, Noris M, De Vriese A, et al. Thrombomodulin mutations in atypical hemolytic-uremic syndrome. N Engl J Med 2009;361(4):345–57.

17. Noris M, Remuzzi G. Atypical hemolytic-uremic syndrome. N Engl J Med 2009; 361(17):1676–87.

18. Kwon T, Dragon-Durey MA, Macher MA, et al. Successful pre-transplant management of a patient with anti-factor H autoantibodies-associated haemolytic uraemic syndrome. Nephrol Dial Transplant 2008;23(6):2088–90.

19. Levi M, Ten Cate H. Disseminated intravascular coagulation. N Engl J Med 1999; 341(8):586–92.

20. Levi M. Current understanding of disseminated intravascular coagulation. Br J Haematol 2004;124(5):567–76.

21. Churchwell KB, McManus ML, Kent P, et al. Intensive blood and plasma exchange for treatment of coagulopathy in meningococcemia. J Clin Apher 1995;10(4):171–7.

22. Niewold TB, Bundrick JB. Disseminated intravascular coagulation due to cytomegalovirus infection in an immunocompetent adult treated with plasma exchange. Am J Hematol 2006;81(6):454–7.

23. Stegmayr BG, Banga R, Berggren L, et al. Plasma exchange as rescue therapy in multiple organ failure including acute renal failure. Crit Care Med 2003;31(6): 1730–6.

24. van Deuren M, Frieling JT, van der Ven-Jongekrijg J, et al. Plasma patterns of tumor necrosis factor-alpha (TNF) and TNF soluble receptors during acute meningococcal infections and the effect of plasma exchange. Clin Infect Dis 1998;26(4):918–23.

25. Nguyen TC, Han YY, Kiss JE, et al. Intensive plasma exchange increases a disintegrin and metalloprotease with thrombospondin motifs-13 activity and reverses organ dysfunction in children with thrombocytopenia-associated multiple organ failure*. Crit Care Med 2008;36(10):2878–87.

26. Nadel S, Goldstein B, Williams MD, et al. Drotrecogin alfa (activated) in children with severe sepsis: a multicentre phase III randomised controlled trial. The Lancet 2007;369(9564):836–43.

27. Asherson RA, Cervera R, de Groot PG, et al. Catastrophic antiphospholipid syndrome: international consensus statement on classification criteria and treatment guidelines. Lupus 2003;12(7):530–4.

28. Cervera R, Font J, Gomez-Puerta JA, et al. Validation of the preliminary criteria for the classification of catastrophic antiphospholipid syndrome. Ann Rheum Dis 2005; 64(8):1205–9.

29. Flamholz R, Tran T, Grad GI, et al. Therapeutic plasma exchange for the acute management of the catastrophic antiphospholipid syndrome: beta(2)-glycoprotein I antibodies as a marker of response to therapy. J Clin Apher 1999;14(4):171–6.

30. Cervera R, Bucciarelli S, Plasin MA, et al. Catastrophic antiphospholipid syndrome (CAPS): descriptive analysis of a series of 280 patients from the "CAPS Registry". J Autoimmun 2009;32(3-4):240–5.

31. Uthman I, Shamseddine A, Taher A. The role of therapeutic plasma exchange in the catastrophic antiphospholipid syndrome. Transfus Apher Sci 2005;33(1):11–7.

32. Ruutu T, Barosi G, Benjamin RJ, et al. Diagnostic criteria for hematopoietic stem cell transplant-associated microangiopathy: results of a consensus process by an International Working Group. Haematologica 2007;92(1):95–100.

33. Uderzo C, Bonanomi S, Busca A, et al. Risk factors and severe outcome in thrombotic microangiopathy after allogeneic hematopoietic stem cell transplantation. Transplantation 2006;82(5):638–44.

34. George JN, Li X, McMinn JR, et al. Thrombotic thrombocytopenic purpura-hemolytic uremic syndrome following allogeneic HPC transplantation: a diagnostic dilemma. Transfusion 2004;44(2):294–304.

35. Elliott MA, Nichols WL Jr, Plumhoff EA, et al. Posttransplantation thrombotic thrombocytopenic purpura: a single-center experience and a contemporary review. Mayo Clin Proc 2003;78(4):421–30.

36. Siami K, Kojouri K, Swisher KK, et al. Thrombotic microangiopathy after allogeneic hematopoietic stem cell transplantation: an autopsy study. Transplantation 2008; 85(1):22–8.

37. Kennedy GA, Kearey N, Bleakley S, et al. Transplantation-associated thrombotic microangiopathy: effect of concomitant GVHD on efficacy of therapeutic plasma exchange. Bone Marrow Transplant 2010;45(4):699–704.

38. Oran B, Donato M, Aleman A, et al. Transplant-associated microangiopathy in patients receiving tacrolimus following allogeneic stem cell transplantation: risk factors and response to treatment. Biol Blood Marrow Transplant 2007;13(4): 469–77.

39. Christidou F, Athanasiadou A, Kalogiannidis P, et al. Therapeutic plasma exchange in patients with grade 2-3 hematopoietic stem cell transplantation-associated thrombotic thrombocytopenic purpura: a ten-year experience. Ther Apher Dial 2003;7(2):259–62.

40. Zakarija A, Kwaan HC, Moake JL, et al. Ticlopidine- and clopidogrel-associated thrombotic thrombocytopenic purpura (TTP): review of clinical, laboratory, epidemiological, and pharmacovigilance findings (1989–2008). Kidney Int Suppl 2009(112): S20–4.

41. Bennett CL, Kim B, Zakarija A, et al. Two mechanistic pathways for thienopyridine-associated thrombotic thrombocytopenic purpura: a report from the SERF-TTP Research Group and the RADAR Project. J Am Coll Cardiol 2007;50(12):1138–43.

42. Naseer N, Aijaz A, Saleem MA, et al. Ticlopidine-associated thrombotic thrombocy-topenic purpura. Heart Dis 2001;3(4):221–3.
43. Pham PT, Peng A, Wilkinson AH, et al. Cyclosporine and tacrolimus-associated thrombotic microangiopathy. Am J Kidney Dis 2000;36(4):844–50.
44. Au WY, Lie AK, Lam CC, et al. Tacrolimus (FK 506) induced thrombotic thrombo-cytopenic purpura after ABO mismatched second liver transplantation: salvage with plasmapheresis and prostacyclin. Haematologica 2000;85(6):659–62.
45. Gupta S, Ttan N, Topolsky D, et al. Thrombotic thrombocytopenic purpura induced by cyclosporin a after allogeneic bone marrow transplantation treated by red blood cell exchange transfusion: a case report. Am J Hematol 2005;80(3):246–7.
46. Nakazawa Y, Hashikura Y, Urata K, et al. Von Willebrand factor–cleaving protease activity in thrombotic microangiopathy after living donor liver transplantation: a case report. Liver Transpl 2003;9(12):1328–33.
47. Bambauer R, Schwarze U, Schiel R. Cyclosporin A and therapeutic plasma ex-change in the treatment of severe systemic lupus erythematosus. Artif Organs 2000;24(11):852–6.
48. Neuwelt CM. The role of plasmapheresis in the treatment of severe central nervous system neuropsychiatric systemic lupus erythematosus. Ther Apher Dial 2003;7(2): 173–82.
49. Schroeder JO, Euler HH. Treatment combining plasmapheresis and pulse cyclo-phosphamide in severe systemic lupus erythematosus. Adv Exp Med Biol 1989;260: 203–13.
50. Canas C, Tobon GJ, Granados M, et al. Diffuse alveolar hemorrhage in Colombian patients with systemic lupus erythematosus. Clin Rheumatol 2007;26(11):1947–9.
51. Wei N, Klippel JH, Huston DP, et al. Randomised trial of plasma exchange in mild systemic lupus erythematosus. Lancet 1983;1(8314–5):17–22.
52. Hanly JG, Hong C, Zayed E, et al. Immunomodulating effects of synchronised plasmapheresis and intravenous bolus cyclophosphamide in systemic lupus ery-thematosus. Lupus 1995;4(6):457–63.
53. Ferenci P. Pathophysiology and clinical features of Wilson disease. Metab Brain Dis 2004;19(3-4):229–39.
54. Asfaha S, Almansori M, Qarni U, et al. Plasmapheresis for hemolytic crisis and impending acute liver failure in Wilson disease. J Clin Apher 2007;22(5):295–8.
55. Hursitoglu M, Kara O, Cikrikcioglu MA, et al. Clinical improvement of a patient with severe Wilson's disease after a single session of therapeutic plasma exchange. J Clin Apher 2009;24(1):25–7.
56. Jhang JS, Schilsky ML, Lefkowitch JH, et al. Therapeutic plasmapheresis as a bridge to liver transplantation in fulminant Wilson disease. J Clin Apher 2007;22(1):10–4.
57. Kiss JE, Berman D, Van Thiel D. Effective removal of copper by plasma exchange in fulminant Wilson's disease. Transfusion 1998;38(4):327–31.
58. Nagata Y, Uto H, Hasuike S, et al. Bridging use of plasma exchange and continuous hemodiafiltration before living donor liver transplantation in fulminant Wilson's dis-ease. Intern Med 2003;42(10):967–70.
59. Lee WM. Acute liver failure. Semin Respir Crit Care Med 2012;33(1):36–45.
60. Clemmesen JO, Kondrup J, Nielsen LB, et al. Effects of high-volume plasmapheresis on ammonia, urea, and amino acids in patients with acute liver failure. Am J Gastroenterol 2001;96(4):1217–23.
61. Ahboucha S, Gamrani H, Baker G. GABAergic neurosteroids: The "endogenous benzodiazepines" of acute liver failure. Neurochem Int 2011. [Epub ahead of print].
62. Akdogan M, Camci C, Gurakar A, et al. The effect of total plasma exchange on fulminant hepatic failure. J Clin Apher 2006;21(2):96–9.

63. De Silvestro G, Marson P, Brandolese R, et al. A single institution's experience (1982–1999) with plasma-exchange therapy in patients with fulminant hepatic failure. Int J Artif Organs 2000;23(7):454–61.

64. Singer AL, Olthoff KM, Kim H, et al. Role of plasmapheresis in the management of acute hepatic failure in children. Ann Surg 2001;234(3):418–24.

65. Rydberg L. ABO-incompatibility in solid organ transplantation. Transfus Med 2001; 11(4):325–42.

66. Roche SL, Burch M, O'Sullivan J, et al. Multicenter experience of ABO-incompatible pediatric cardiac transplantation. Am J Transplant 2008;8(1):208–15.

67. West LJ, Pollock-Barziv SM, Dipchand AI, et al. ABO-incompatible heart transplantation in infants. N Engl J Med 2001;344(11):793–800.

68. Carithers RL Jr. Liver transplantation. American Association for the Study of Liver Diseases. Liver Transpl 2000;6(1):122–35.

69. Winters JL, Gloor JM, Pineda AA, et al. Plasma exchange conditioning for ABO-incompatible renal transplantation. J Clin Apher 2004;19(2):79–85.

70. Tobian AA, Shirey RS, Montgomery RA, et al. Therapeutic plasma exchange reduces ABO titers to permit ABO-incompatible renal transplantation. Transfusion 2009; 49(6):1248–54.

71. Khurana DS, Melvin JJ, Kothare SV, et al. Acute disseminated encephalomyelitis in children: discordant neurologic and neuroimaging abnormalities and response to plasmapheresis. Pediatrics 2005;116(2):431–6.

72. Lin CH, Jeng JS, Yip PK. Plasmapheresis in acute disseminated encephalomyelitis. J Clin Apher 2004;19(3):154–9.

73. RamachandranNair R, Rafeequ M, Girija AS. Plasmapheresis in childhood acute disseminated encephalomyelitis. Indian Pediatr 2005;42(5):479–82.

74. Garg RK. Acute disseminated encephalomyelitis. Postgrad Med J 2003;79(927): 11–7.

75. Kaynar L, Altuntas F, Aydogdu I, et al. Therapeutic plasma exchange in patients with neurologic diseases: retrospective multicenter study. Transfus Apher Sci 2008; 38(2):109–15.

76. Keegan M, Pineda AA, McClelland RL, et al. Plasma exchange for severe attacks of CNS demyelination: predictors of response. Neurology 2002;58(1):143–6.

77. Menge T, Hemmer B, Nessler S, et al. Acute disseminated encephalomyelitis: an update. Arch Neurol 2005;62(11):1673–80.

78. Johnson JP, Moore J Jr, Austin HA 3rd, et al. Therapy of anti-glomerular basement membrane antibody disease: analysis of prognostic significance of clinical, pathologic and treatment factors. Medicine (Baltimore) 1985;64(4):219–27.

79. Levy JB, Turner AN, Rees AJ, et al. Long-term outcome of anti-glomerular basement membrane antibody disease treated with plasma exchange and immunosuppression. Ann Intern Med 2001;134(11):1033–42.

80. Simpson IJ, Doak PB, Williams LC, et al. Plasma exchange in Goodpasture's syndrome. Am J Nephrol 1982;2(6):301–11.

81. Lazor R, Bigay-Game L, Cottin V, et al. Alveolar hemorrhage in anti-basement membrane antibody disease: a series of 28 cases. Medicine (Baltimore) 2007;86(3): 181–93.

82. Zauner I, Bach D, Braun N, et al. Predictive value of initial histology and effect of plasmapheresis on long-term prognosis of rapidly progressive glomerulonephritis. Am J Kidney Dis 2002;39(1):28–35.

83. Little MA, Pusey CD. Rapidly progressive glomerulonephritis: current and evolving treatment strategies. J Nephrol 2004;17(Suppl 8):S10–9.

84. Frasca GM, Soverini ML, Falaschini A, et al. Plasma exchange treatment improves prognosis of antineutrophil cytoplasmic antibody-associated crescentic glomerulonephritis: a case-control study in 26 patients from a single center. Ther Apher Dial 2003;7(6):540–6.

85. Klemmer PJ, Chalermskulrat W, Reif MS, et al. Plasmapheresis therapy for diffuse alveolar hemorrhage in patients with small-vessel vasculitis. Am J Kidney Dis 2003;42(6):1149–53.

86. de Lind van Wijngaarden RA, Hauer HA, Wolterbeek R, et al. Clinical and histologic determinants of renal outcome in ANCA-associated vasculitis: a prospective analysis of 100 patients with severe renal involvement. J Am Soc Nephrol 2006;17(8):2264–74.

87. Jayne DR, Gaskin G, Rasmussen N, et al. Randomized trial of plasma exchange or high-dosage methylprednisolone as adjunctive therapy for severe renal vasculitis. J Am Soc Nephrol 2007;18(7):2180–8.

88. Henter JI, Horne A, Arico M, et al. HLH-2004: Diagnostic and therapeutic guidelines for hemophagocytic lymphohistiocytosis. Pediatr Blood Cancer 2007; 48(2):124–31.

89. Jordan MB, Allen CE, Weitzman S, et al. How I treat hemophagocytic lymphohistiocytosis. Blood 2011;118(15):4041–52.

90. Castillo L, Carcillo J. Secondary hemophagocytic lymphohistiocytosis and severe sepsis/systemic inflammatory response syndrome/multiorgan dysfunction syndrome/macrophage activation syndrome share common intermediate phenotypes on a spectrum of inflammation. Pediatr Crit Care Med 2009;10(3): 387–92.

91. Coman T, Dalloz MA, Coolen N, et al. Plasmapheresis for the treatment of acute pancreatitis induced by hemophagocytic syndrome related to hypertriglyceridemia. J Clin Apher 2003;18(3):129–31.

92. Imashuku S, Hibi S, Ohara T, et al. Effective control of Epstein-Barr virus-related hemophagocytic lymphohistiocytosis with immunochemotherapy. Histiocyte Society. Blood 1999;93(6):1869–74.

93. Ladisch S, Ho W, Matheson D, et al. Immunologic and clinical effects of repeated blood exchange in familial erythrophagocytic lymphohistiocytosis. Blood 1982;60(4): 814–21.

94. Nakakura H, Ashida A, Matsumura H, et al. A case report of successful treatment with plasma exchange for hemophagocytic syndrome associated with severe systemic juvenile idiopathic arthritis in an infant girl. Ther Apher Dial 2009;13(1): 71–6.

95. Raschke RA, Garcia-Orr R. Hemophagocytic lymphohistiocytosis: a potentially underrecognized association with systemic inflammatory response syndrome, severe sepsis, and septic shock in adults. Chest 2011;140(4):933–8.

96. Sanada S, Ookawara S, Shindo T, et al. A case report of the effect of plasma exchange on reactive hemophagocytic syndrome associated with toxic shock syndrome. Ther Apher Dial 2004;8(6):503–6.

97. Satomi A, Nagai S, Nagai T, et al. Effect of plasma exchange on refractory hemophagocytic syndrome complicated with myelodysplastic syndrome. Ther Apher 1999;3(4):317–9.

98. Song KS, Sung HJ. Effect of plasma exchange on the circulating IL-6 levels in a patient with fatal hemophagocytic syndrome associated with bile ductopenia. Ther Apher Dial 2006;10(1):87–9.

99. Zhang XY, Ye XW, Feng DX, et al. Hemophagocytic lymphohistiocytosis induced by severe pandemic influenza A (H1N1) 2009 virus infection: a case report. Case Report Med 2011;2011:951910.

100. Demirkol D, Yildizdas D, Bayrakci B, et al. Hyperferritinemia in the critically ill child with secondary HLH/sepsis/MODS/MAS: what is the treatment? Crit Care 2012; 16(2):R52.

# Index

*Note:* Page numbers of article titles are in **boldface** type.

## A

Acute lung injury (ALI)
    transfusion-related, **363–372**. *See also* Transfusion-related acute lung injury (TRALI)
ALI. *See* Acute lung injury (ALI)
Anemia
    described, 345–346
    in ICU, **333–343**
        epidemiology of, 333–334
        severity of, 346
        treatment of, 340–342
            EPO in, 350–357
            erythropoietic agents in, 341
            hepcidin antagonists in, 342
            iron therapy in, 341–342
            red cell transfusions in, 340–341
    of inflammation
        described, 338
        in ICU .
            with concurrent iron deficiency, 338–339
            pathophysiology of, 334–338
                described, 334–335
                genes involved in hepcidin regulation in, 338
                iron absorption in, 335–336
                iron homeostasis regulation in, 336–338
                iron transport and storage in, 336
    predilection for, 346
    prevalence of, 345–346
Anti-Xa inhibitors
    indirect
        in critically ill patients
            pharmacology and evidence from clinical trials, 430–431
Anticoagulant(s)
    newer agents
        in critically ill patients, **427–451**
            bleeding due to
                management of, 443–444
            indirect anti-Xa inhibitors
                overdosing/underdosing of, 442
            LMWHs
                overdosing/underdosing of, 441–443

Crit Care Clin 28 (2012) 469–478
http://dx.doi.org/10.1016/S0749-0704(12)00046-2
0749-0704/12/$ – see front matter © 2012 Elsevier Inc. All rights reserved.

criticalcare.theclinics.com

# Moving?

## Make sure your subscription moves with you!

To notify us of your new address, find your **Clinics Account Number** (located on your mailing label above your name), and contact customer service at:

**Email: journalscustomerservice-usa@elsevier.com**

**800-654-2452** (subscribers in the U.S. & Canada)
**314-447-8871** (subscribers outside of the U.S. & Canada)

**Fax number: 314-447-8029**

**Elsevier Health Sciences Division**
**Subscription Customer Service**
**3251 Riverport Lane**
**Maryland Heights, MO 63043**

*To ensure uninterrupted delivery of your subscription, please notify us at least 4 weeks in advance of move.

Printed and bound by CPI Group (UK) Ltd, Croydon, CR0 4YY

13/10/2024

01773590-0003